EARTH CAN BE A LONELY PLACE.

Various Authors

First published April 2020
ISBN: 9798851385254

Edited by Meek © 2020
Front cover Artwork Stephen Scott © 2020

An Amazon KDP Publication ©2020

Foreword

This was put together during springtime in 2020, for future generations – yes this did occur. It brought earth's inhabitants to a standstill. It changed our lives forever. What you're about receive are snapshots of our existence.

Meek on behalf of the authors.
2020.

Disclaimer of Liability
The material contained in this book is the personal views of the authors and contributors. You should not rely upon the contents as advice or information or as a basis for making any legal or medical decisions.

For

Gaia.

From the Greek word γαια (Gaia), a parallel form of γη (ge) meaning "earth". In Greek mythology Gaia was the mother goddess who presided over the earth. She was the mate of Uranus and the mother of the Titans and the Cyclopes.

"Don't Worry, Grandma, I'll be better in no time and this virus will be chucked out to space soon."

Zac Noah McIntosh (Aged 5 years old)

EARTH
CAN
BE
A
LONELY
PLACE

Authors & Contributors

Andy Greenhouse, Meek, Alex Main, Heidi Kaplan,
George Colkitto, Jimmy Kellock, Pamela Borland,
Christine Tait, Becca Mascull, Brian McNee,
Rosemary Bird, Mo Scott, Audrey Keenan, Neil MacLean,
Davy Craig, Derek B Steel, Leela Soma, Cat Corbally,
Carol Allan, Jim MacKellar, Davy Craig, Tyhe Paul Egar,
Maliny van der Mysteries, Alex Hughes, Michelle Carr,
Katrina McKeown, Erik Zoha, Paul Gallagher, Sue Cooper,
Ali Paterson Archer, Lorna Kerr, Rosetta Muscatt,
Amanda Austin, Ross Wilcock, Kelly Greenhouse,
Jon Bickley, Anon, James Molloy,
John Roche, Dougie Smith, Sean Conroy, Doug Molloy,
Scott Steel, Janette Fenton, Fee Johnstone, Alex Hastings,
John Innes, Scott McKinlay, James Barney Ward,
Tohm Bakelas, Jackie Reilly, Mr Hemp, Janet Crawford,
Andy Gee, Dave Jay Coutts, Neil Hodge,
Dr Ian Mowbray, Sandra Alexander, Michael Zur-Szpiro,
Simon Rowberry, Jessica Allan, Lynn Ainslie, Andrea Doria,
Stephen Scott, Niamh Mahon.

Contents —

Today Should Have Been.

Today should have been day 2 of our adventure to Tenerife
for a cheeky cheap and cheerful holiday to get away from
the winter blues and recharge our souls. Last holiday we had
was six months ago in September... but, as we all know only
too well, the whole world has come crashing down around
us and I know that our paltry little cancelled weeks holiday
in the sun is nothing in comparison to some of the heartbreak
that people have had to endure because of this fucking virus
but. Everything matters in its own way... so I got to thinking.
what would we have been doing right now if we had indeed
got to Las Galletas in Tenerife... and I'd like to think it might
have   been   something   like   this...

altered   reality

In an alternative universe where hand gel hardens in disused
bottles
and mountains of luxurious tissue paper disintegrate into dust
where   crowds   congregate   oblivious   of   any   Covid-19
catastrophe
I went for a stroll with my loved one intent on a seafood
dinner

the evening was balmy and just right for flip-flops shorts
and   a   tee
though she of course wore that floral summer dress just
above   her   knee

and we walked hand in hand along white tiled Calle
pavements
to the cacophonic accompaniment of countless Canarian
cicadae

at a charming taverna on the marina promenade we arrived
and gazed at the voluminous fish tank in which lobsters with
taped up pincers fretted in anticipation of selection while
friendly waiters urged us in with tired clichés as we studied
the   menu

he told us his name was Miguel as he showed us to a table
under   a   straw
canopy from where we could watch the yachts and fishing
skiffs   as   they
came and went from the small harbour with their lights
twinkling   in   the   dusk
and their wakes causing the moored boats to rise and bob
against   the   jetty

he left us with the menu but quickly returned with olives and
bread   and   oil
and a jug of water which we politely declined and asked for
baileys   and   wine
and again he left us with si senor but not before lighting a
candle   stump   which
gave off a sweet scent and spluttered as a mosquito got too
close   and   ignited

the rickety table was covered by a worn plastic tablecloth
with a pattern of shells
across which we held hands as we waited patiently for our
order to materialise
my dish of grilled octopus on a bed of sautéed potato slices
with garlic was
sublime whilst Wendy claimed her calamari was the best
she'd ever tasted

and while we ate we talked and reminisced of all the meals
we'd eaten like this
and considered and gave thanks at how lucky we were to
have the opportunity
to travel and enjoy the fruits of our labours and the freedom
that foreign holidays
give us and we asked Miguel to take a picture of us and left
him a big tip

we walked back to the hotel up through the old town and
stopped at a noisy bar
with a chalkboard outside that proclaimed happy hour eight
til midnight and karaoke
so of course we had to go in for a nightcap and maybe to
sing a song or two to the
babbling crowd that was a good mixture of nationalities all
enjoying a good time

we stumbled our way home and finally made it back to the
hotel at almost two am

tripping through the front door across the deserted foyer and
up   the   stairs   to   our   room
which we found eventually although we struggled to get the
electronic   lock   to   open
but we got in and made coffee in the kitchen and love on the
balcony   and   fell   asleep   by   three

tomorrow we shall likely have a holiday hangover which
shall   be   cured   by   bacon
and we might go for a walk along the playa or lounge in the
sun   by   the   seawater   pool
for this is the life we all should lead instead of this altered
reality   of   broken   dreams
that we now suffer in the isolatory abandonment of a novel
corona nightmare.

Andy Greenhouse.
29.03.20

Self-Isolation #1.

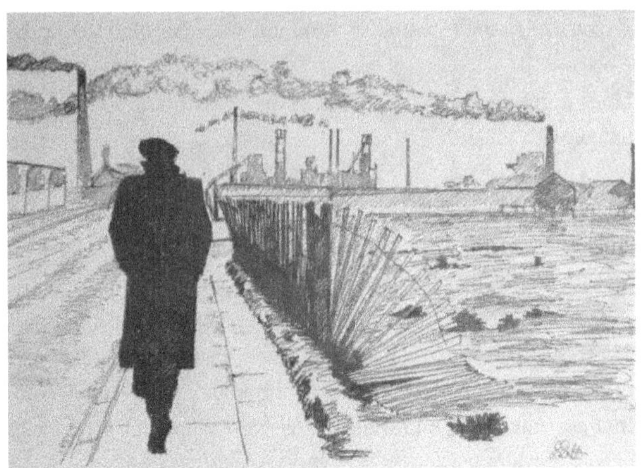

Stephen Scott.

Self-Isolation #2.

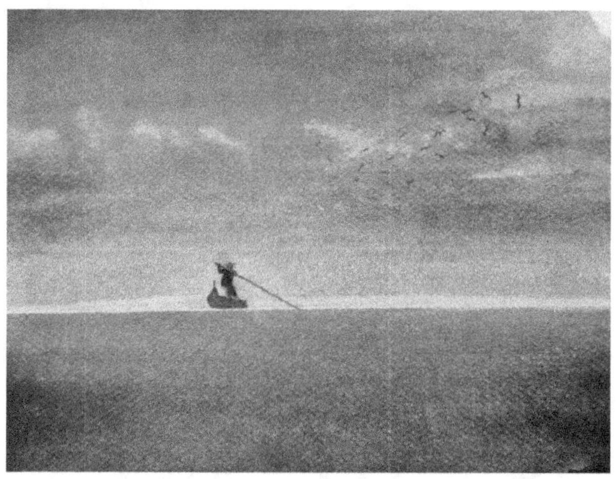

Stephen Scott.

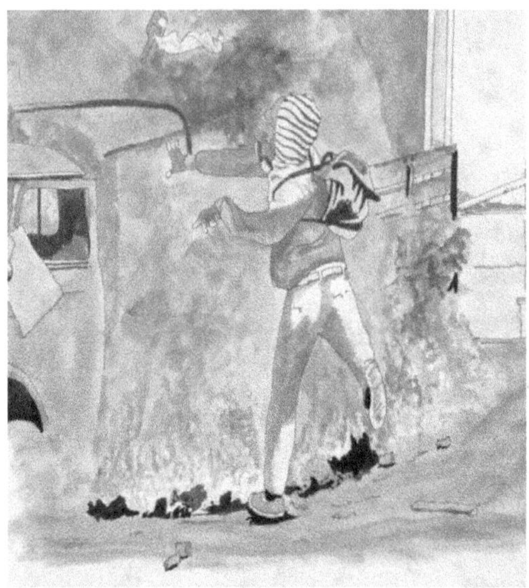

Stephen Scott.

Stay Safe.

- Take two paracetamol
- I'm allergic to them
- Take two paracetamol and self-isolate
- But I'm allergic to them and I get lonely
- You can Skype someone, a member of your family or a friend
- I'm not close to my family and don't keep in touch with any friends
- You could read a book or watch a programme or listen to the radio
- I've got a short attention span, and to be honest I'm what you'd call illiterate
- You need to self-isolate, quarantine yourself
- I'm already in quarantine. I live alone. I don't see anyone from day to day.

Quarantine

/ˈkwɒrəntiːn/
Learn to pronounce

Noun

noun: quarantine; plural noun: quarantines
a state, period, or place of isolation in which people or animals that have arrived from elsewhere or been exposed to infectious or contagious disease are placed.
"many animals die in quarantine"

Verb

verb: quarantine; 3rd person present: quarantines; past tense:
quarantined; past participle: quarantined; gerund or present
participle: quarantining
put (a person or animal) in quarantine.
"I quarantine all new fish for one month"
Origin

mid-17th century: from Italian quarantina 'forty days', from
quaranta 'forty'.

- But what do you mean?
- Take two paracetamol and keep away from
  everyone else for a fortnight, two weeks, minimum
- I'm allergic to paracetamol, they upset my stomach
- Well it's either that or a possibility of you dying or
  passing the virus onto others. That would be
  irresponsible now wouldn't it? You don't want to
  infect others, possibly kill them, be responsible for
  their deaths now do you?

Death

/dɛθ/
Learn to pronounce

Noun

noun: death; plural noun: deaths

the action or fact of dying or being killed; the end of the life of a
person or organism.
"he had been depressed since the death of his father"
Similar:
demise
dying
end
passing
passing away
passing on
loss of life
expiry
expiration
departure from life
final exit
eternal rest
murder
killing
assassination
execution
dispatch
slaying
slaughter
massacre
snuffing
curtains
kicking the bucket
decease
quietus

Opposite:

life
the state of being dead.

"even in death, she was beautiful"
the permanent ending of vital processes in a cell or tissue.
the personification of the power that destroys life, often represented
in art and literature as a skeleton or an old man holding a scythe.

Noun: Death

Similar:
the Grim Reaper
the Dark Angel
the Angel of Death
the destruction or permanent end of something.
"the death of her hopes"
Similar:
end
finish
cessation
termination
extinction
extinguishing
collapse
ruin
ruination
destruction
extermination
eradication
annihilation
obliteration
extirpation

Opposite:
birth
a damaging or destructive state of affairs.
"to be driven to a dance by one's father would be social death"

- No, you're right; I don't want that on my conscience.
  But I am allergic to paracetamol, and I don't much
  like any foreign substances entering my body. I
  don't like the feelings. The anti-depressants are bad
  enough. How come you think that there's always a
  magic pill, a cure-all, a panacea?
- Look, it's entirely up to you. This is my professional
  advice. Take two paracetamol and isolate yourself
  for two weeks at least. The sooner you do this the
  sooner you'll get back to normal. And you'll be
  helping yourself, your community, this country, and
  the world in general on the road to recovery.
- But I don't really have a high temperature or a
  fever. I've got a sore throat, feel nauseous, and I
  hear buzz-saw noises in my head.
- Have you had any more thoughts about self-
  harming?
- Yeah. All the time. Every second of every hour of
  the day, every day of the week.

Self-harm

/sɛlfˈhɑːm/

Verb

gerund or present participle: self-harming
commit self-harm.

Self-harm is when somebody intentionally damages or injures their
body. It's usually a way of coping with or expressing overwhelming
emotional distress.

Self-harm, also known as self-injury, is defined as the intentional, direct injuring of body tissue, done without the intent to commit suicide. Other terms such as...

- (Fuxake. It's a bad day for humans when Wikifuckedia has a definition for my condition.)
- What thoughts are you harbouring?
- Still the bridge, visiting the bridge. A specific spot, an exact location
- Have you spoken to anyone else about this
- No, not yet
- Are you like to act on these thoughts
- I don't know. I really don't know
- Thanks for sharing this with me
- It was kinda difficult, you know
- Oh, I appreciate that. Are you still carrying a rope around with you
- Not so much these days

Bridge

/brɪdʒ/
See definitions in:
All
Civil Engineering
Transportation
Anatomy
Dentistry
Music
Billiards
Electrical

Noun

1.

a structure carrying a road, path, railway, etc. across a river, road,
or other obstacle.
"a bridge across the River Thames"
Similar:
viaduct
aqueduct
flyover
overpass
way over

2.

the elevated, enclosed platform on a ship from which the captain
and officers direct operations.
"Talbot stepped across the two gunwales and made his way up to
the bridge"

Verb

be or make a bridge over (something).
"a covered walkway bridged the gardens"
Similar:
span
cross
cross over
go over
pass over
extend across
reach across
traverse

-     And what was the plan with the rope
-     To find a secluded spot. Isn't it healthy to flirt with
      these thoughts and to test resolve

Flirt

/flə:t/
Learn to pronounce

Verb
1.
behave as though sexually attracted to someone, but playfully rather
than with serious intentions.
"she began to tease him, flirting with other men in front of him"
Similar:
trifle with
toy with
tease
lead on
philander with
dally with
make romantic advances to
court
woo
vamp
pull
chat up
make eyes at
make sheep's eyes at
give the come-on to
come on to
be all over
set one's cap at

2.
(of a bird) wave or open and shut (its wings or tail) with a quick
flicking motion.
"a moorhen stepped out of the reeds, flirting its white tail"

Noun
a person who habitually flirts.
"Jim was an outrageous flirt"
Similar:
tease
trifler
philanderer
coquette
heartbreaker
puss
ladies' man
fizgig
gallant
vulgar slangcock-teaser

- (The only thing I can relate to above, as a meaning

   is — *Vulgar Slangcock Teaser)*

- How do you mean — test your resolve

- By testing myself. To see if I'm brave or a coward.

   Bravery or cowardice. If I act upon these feelings

   am I brave for doing so or a coward for not

- I've never heard of that before.

- It's new to me as well

- You must try to get more exercise, and socialise.

  You need to get out more

- But you said self-isolate. I don't get endorphins, or

  any energy rush. Nothing stirs me. Everything's an

  effort.

- Take two paracetamol

- But I'm allergic.

Meek.
March 2020.

The Small Bottle.

The small bottle arrived as an offering from the sea to the land.
It was carried on the back of a wave that whispered a kiss as it touched the sand warmed by the sun.
Light danced off the surface of its blue glass and caught the attention of a small child who was digging holes for no other reason than she could.
Rescuing it from the next wave that threatened to snatch it quickly back she held it in her hand and marvelled at the swirling contents.
Older eyes would have no doubt described what they seen within as the chaos of the universe as it seemed that tiny stars were continuously exploding and birthing smaller planets, but for the child only one word could cover what she could see, and that was magic.
Holding it aloft ever more colours came to life and the temptation to pull the cork from the bottle and pour a little on her hand became a temptation that couldn't be denied.
The cork stopper slid from the bottle with no effort and with it she heard a soft pop.
With that pop she blinked and in the fraction of the second of her eyelids closing and opening again there stood a man.
A giant of a man.
A man wearing a suit that reminded her of the plumage of exotic birds that she had always seen in books, but never up close.

He smiled and she felt instantly calm as he knelt before her
so that they faced each other as equals.
In a voice that she heard only in her head he asked her if
she knew what a wish was.
She looked into his eyes and seen that they were shining
with the contents of the little bottle and in a clear voice she
said that she did.
A moment passed and his voice then asked her if she wanted
one, but only one.
Without breaking eye contact she replied 'yes, yes I do'.
Reaching out he then placed his hands on her shoulders and
she heard his voice say to her to let her heart speak.
And she did.
She wished for love.
It was a simple wish, but a far reaching one. A child's
understanding of love is uncorrupted. It is imbued with
kindness, compassion and natural empathy.
This was her wish.
The man rose and looked to the sea and then to the sky and
then to the land and whispered aloud 'as it shall it be.'
And it was.
From where they stood at the edge of the sea the wish
rippled out and enveloped the world.
No one really knew why, but while anger was remembered
no one felt any in themselves anymore.
Fists unclenched, weapons were set aside, words of hate were
left unsaid and instead everyone seen each other as true
family. Every father was a father to all. Every mother a
mother to all. Every woman a sister. Every man a brother.

Kneeling back down the man held out his hand and in it was
the little glass bottle, and with a blink from the little girl she
was looking at it in her own hand.
She smiled. It felt different now. Lighter.
Instinctually she knew that she couldn't keep it and with as
much strength as she had in her tiny body she threw it as
far as she could back into the sea.
Turning she looked up the beach to see her mother and
father walking hand in hand towards her.
Running towards them she threw herself into her mother's
arms and was swung up onto her father's shoulders.
I love you she said.
Of course you do. Everyone loves everyone don't they.
And she knew that they did.

Alex Main.

Coming In Blue.

My time is coming
I've had enough of this shit
I will be free and single
Not attached like a stone

I will sing triumphantly
I've served my sentence now
I choose life as the t shirt said
Not hard labour

I've weathered a storm
Where nobody else got wet
They won't go when I go
Mr Stevie wonder poetically said

I have only two purposes
To laugh and to love
And to be loved in return

I feel worn out
Like an old pair of shoes
I'll sit here and rest
And write away the coming in blue

Heidi Kaplan.

Two Poems from Lockdown – Day 14

Eton Boy.

do you want to destroy a life
clip the wings
it's not just the control
it's the loss of flight
never to see from above
how the world stretches
limitless

you want to destroy a life
say this is where you stay
in these meagre days
here in the strife and rubble
trachled in glaur
there is no dream to soar
the reality of birth

George Colkitto. March 2020.

Hope.

tomorrow I may be someone new
as if I was not who I am
tomorrow another vision
I can walk to anywhere
pretend yesterday was a lie
become taller and clever
how long can I hold on today
discover the night

yesterday is old
eat my chips
throw away the paper

today
                cry
                                  fail

succeed

                      sing

George Colkitto. March 2020

1914 – 2020.

1914
"Your Country Needs You"
To fuckin' die
2020
"Your Country Needs You"
To Fuckin' die
Fooled Again
By Money Junkies
With their Non-Elected
Backroom Flunkies
There is no money
In this country
No Protection
For The Monkeys
Then out pops
A money tree
The Likes of which
We've never seen
Where the fuck
Has it all been
For Decades
It's Just Obscene
Handing cash
Out to the masses
Don't Forget The
Middle Classes
They're always there

The bigot fascists
Making Moves
With Square Moustaches
It's all big business
In the end
They Don't like you
You're no friend
Wear Your masks
Until the end
Poor Bastards
Will You Ever Learn
Goodbye Freedom
Goodbye Hope
Let's See These Despots
On A Rope
They Don't Fool Me
With Bars Of Soap
I Have Green
And I Will Cope

Jimmy Kellock.

Hmm, I'll Try.

Hmmm, I'll try,
What about though? Head Birling with crap but wouldn't know where to start
What about my Son in lockdown 2020, his devotion and Passion for his garden?
Making lockdown pleasant to look at and how it's actually Slowing us and the world down,
To repair itself, give us time to think of all the things we Actually took for granted,
Like just jumping to the shop without a queue, not having to Wash your hands at every opportunity till they bleed,
Not having to stand in lengthy queues for meds at chemist And the government not giving our NHS proper PPE to wear...
I could go on but the positive for me is my son and nature.

Pamela Borland.
March 2020.

Mother Nature's Tarot Reading.

The graveyard of Eden
Mother Nature's tarot reading
The sewers haemorrhage
Sticky seas of porridge

The city has no pulse
It danced the last waltz
Exhaust pipes with siren bells
Like bats out of hell

Horns bark thirteen o'clock
Creatures in states of shock
Clumsy and concussed
Fields are toasted crusts

Fossils eclipse rubble
Jungle fluff and stubble
Smoulder like a grill
Swamps froth flasks of krill

Rivers lethal tonic
Decay so crude and chronic
Gremlin's septic cocktails
Of dodos, mammoths and whales

The chemical picnics
Forests are stilts and sticks
A spiralling headline
To earth's beckoning deadline

Thank you. Kind regards. Chris

Christine Tait.

Maliny van der Mysteries Sent Me A Video.

Maliny sent me a video as an attachment
Which I couldn't include in this book
Its content was informative, it was insightful
It was just, and it was poetic
I apologised
But it was a video nonetheless.

Meek.

Not A Good Day Yesterday.

Not a good day yesterday.
Felt like my brain was turning to mush.
Could take no pleasure in anything.
Irritable and depressed. Stir crazy.
Worst day yet, I'd say.
But I feel brighter this morning.
I'm going to try to write a chapter today, to feel some progress in something.
I think it hit me this is not going to change anytime soon, so I need to accept this as the new normal.
How are you guys doing?

Becca Mascull.

3 Photographs From Ash.

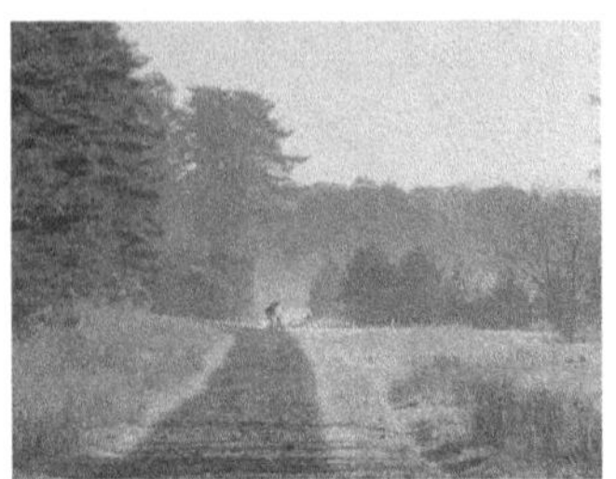

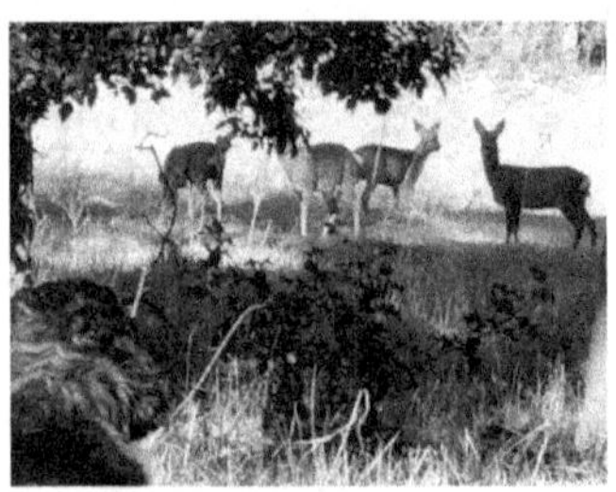

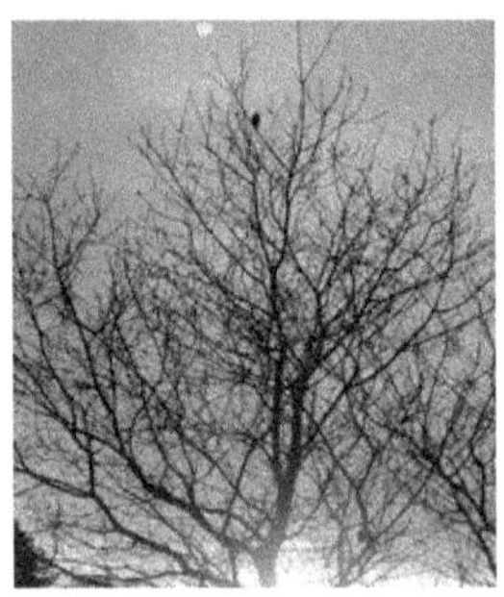

Ash J. Farraway.

Family Values.

Gone are the days of the old Butt and Ben
We're long past the age of the wee single end
Modern houses are built with bathrooms to spare
Thrown up by planners with barely a care

So as rooms increase in their number and size
The family unit begins its demise
Kids go to their rooms, barely a teen
Then six long years later, return moody and mean

I sit down the stairs with a glass in my hand
Penning a poem you may not understand
Mum's in her bed, watching TV
Kids in their own world, leaving one lonely me

My music's a mixture of The Doors and Pink Floyd
Reviving some memories, I'd rather avoid
One minute it inspires, the next I'm so sad
And this is the point, I get pretty mad

The family unit, its values dismissed
My whisky in hand, as I get slowly pissed
How can I be lonely, with so many around?
Just ten feet away, but nowhere to be found!

I think of some friends, and think "how do they cope"?
And the fact that they do, fills me with hope
My loneliness dwarfed, by the burden they bear
I send them my love, and hope they know that I care

So I'll sit here and listen to my music of old
I'll keep my chin up, and try to be bold
Family values should be held close and dear
Hold on to your loved ones and make your love clear.

Brian McNee.

Two Wolves

There once lived wise old Indian chief
Known for his calm nature and sage
One day he's approached by a young angry buck
Known for his temper and rage

"I see from your eyes, torture grips at your soul"
Whispers the chief to this unsteady foul
"Oh chief I'm so frightened by the thoughts in my head"
One moment I'm happy, the next I wish me dead"

The chief rests a grizzled hand on the shoulder of his ward
"One day you reach for flowers, the next you reach for
sword"?
"My boy, within us all, there lives two Wolves who fight"
"One wolf is full of darkness, the other full of light"

"But chief, then who determines my soul's eventual path"?
"I fear not for me, but for the tribe, as I am so full of wrath "
The chief's hand rests so gently, on the shoulder that is bare
Whilst his other hand now tussles the young buck's long dark
hair

"Listen very closely, for what I say is true"
"To ignore these words could be the end of all that's good in
you"

"We all face this dilemma, no matter what our creed"
"The wolf who wins the battle is the very wolf we feed."

Brian McNee.

And 1 For The kids:

Sweet Dreams.

When I was a baby, I once had a dream
About mountains of chocolate, and rivers of cream
With steps made of biscuit, that reach to the sky
And all the cars wheels are hot apple pie

The flowers are puff candy, with liquorish stalks
And chocolate buttons, adorn ladies frocks
With grass of green fondant, all springy and soft
And lawnmowers are people, who live on a croft

There are clouds of marshmallow, and snowdrops are sweets
That fall down as showers, on caramel streets
With massive volcanoes of sweet candy floss
Streaming with lava, of hot chocolate sauce

Where strawberry cats, chase white chocolate mice
Across lakes of treacle, and puddles of rice
Now I'm a bit older, I still close my eyes
And hope for my dream, of blueberry skies.

Brian McNee.

Rosemary Forwarded A Photograph.

*Today is the
world "Close
Friend Day"
Send this to your
friends, even
me- if I'm one of
them. See how
many you get! I
hope you get a
dozen!*

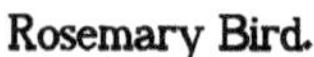

Rosemary Bird.

Aye ... Think That's Why I Like Yer Work.

I've always written; as a wee girl I spent a lot of time on my own either in hospital or at home. Writing, drawing, reading and taking apart watches and clocks ...😊 😁

Music was always huge for us. My huge family in Helensburgh were a great influence. My Daddy was a Minstrel, back in the day ' black face ' was considered normal (ugh) ...his sisters entertained in the 'Honky Tonk' dancehall. His Daddy played banjo, his brother the piano. My Dad used to practice his harmonica listening to very old records. Daddy once stole a Saxophone out of Taylor's music shop in an effort to upgrade. He did the crime, but his wee brother got lifted for it, they looked like twins ...my sweet wee uncle Goo was known to be a bit light of the finger, he did the time and never grassed my Daddy up.... Dunno if there was a piano in the bad boys' school ... Family ties!

My Mum was from an Irish family and Grandpa Lolly played fiddle. My Mum played piano. The musical gene passed me by, but not my love of it. It's the breath of life.

I was delighted when my son took up guitar, started a band and for 18 years stuck with it. 'The Devotions ' ' The Elvis Suicide ' and CDEX (Chris Devotion and the Expectations). He can play guitar, banjo mandolin and a wee bit piano, not a bad singer either. We are all sad that stopped. So now he does improv and stand up.

My writing has continued, though when Scotty and I started art classes and I found colour, the painting took over. Apart from a few poems published in those Poetry Now anthologies.

I've never pursued it.
I need to get through my notebooks.
I find your poems always rhythmic, surprising and thought provoking. Just like good music.

Now I have to be even more careful... Winters are crap for my heart and lungs. Spring is my rebirth! ... Thankfully we have a garden and the Forth and Clyde canal at the end of the road.

The Ducks like a bit of Tamla Motown...though they bugger off sharpish when I let rip wi' Iggy and the Stooges.

Canny please everyone eh...
You take care, and keep the joy comin'

Singing is braw for the lungs and I'm thinking the Harmonica might be a go-er for lung function...

Mo Scott.

Found Their Inner Angel And Shared.

The end was just the beginning....
They thought they had lost. But they were winning. Staying home in solitude only did the mind some good. Being more creative realising the meaning of life. Mortality remembering those who have a place in our heart. Feeling sad that we could possibly part. Appreciating all that we may have taken for granted. Awakening to a new earth. One that humans didn't judge, really cared. Loving more, found their inner angel and shared.

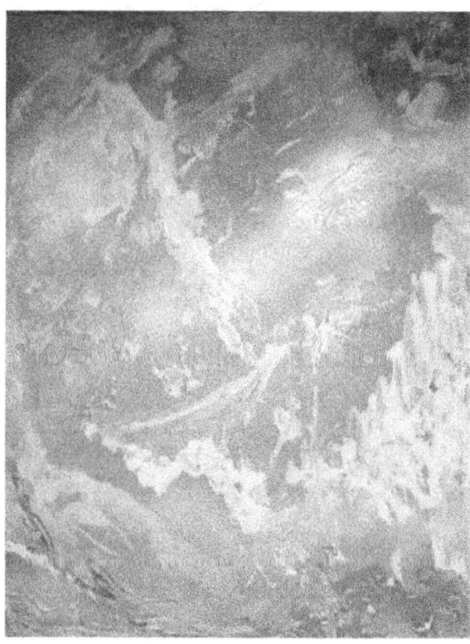

Audrey Keenan.

And A Light Sister.

Why do we even need money when humanity can come together and solve and fix some if not most of its underlying issues and ills of the world, through a virus just because it shows no borders and that it can effect anyone so some people will and eventually wake up too their spell bound realities as well as lifestyles that some have been under that does it all really matter in the bigger scheme of things. So a good majority of it when it wishes too pulls together can really show us all what it's really capable of with positive & humanistic mind set with no one particular person gaining from it mostly. So only if humanity is allowed to do so without certain others getting in its way at times, as it does so from time to time, society can always overcome, whom as well as making and creating situations deliberately or unknowingly for something that the world calls money too which can lead to manifesting more negative energy from us to control each individual desires for material items for a minority to mostly gain from which don't even require or need though it can and should be shared for all and everyone needs and aspirations for a more healthy and environmentally better world to live in and move into higher dimensions within the universe if done so. Hope you well M sending you and the family ♥ □ and light sister x

Neil MacLean.

Lockdown.

Life doesn't seem to be all that different to me.
Having been isolated for the last six years.
I'd only just started going out, you see
And starting to face many of my fears.

I'm physically disabled, with a knackered back
And a gammy knee from a crash.
I'd been trying to get my life on track,
But depression could appear in a flash.

I finished therapy and was ready for it
It certainly helped in a positive way
I was fed up of just having to sit
Alone, so started to get out each day.

I stuttered my way through a course enrolment
For anxiety, through talking face to face.
It all helped to halt my rapid descent
Into a much deeper and darker place.

Life started to have some purpose and I was feeling better
A sense of wellbeing purveyed
Then the virus arrived like a DWP letter
Unwelcome, invasive, making so many afraid.

I worry for others around the world
In this time that'll go down in folklore
wondering how this scenario will unfold
Asking questions: How? why? and what for?

I'm not alone all day, like I was in the past
I have my partner and son to keep me sane,
But what makes it all worse is the stark contrast
Of others stuck in by themselves and in pain.

Many live like this every day of the year
And struggle to cope at the best of times
with no one around to hold them dear
I'm thankful for all that I have, sometimes.

I try to joke and write daft stories
It helps to keep in touch
Telling tales of the past, reliving past glories
with old pals, there with just one touch.

People mention the wars and of heroes past
But the legends of today are nurses and docs
And others who always put themselves last,
Providing us all with a future beyond this pox.

They all deserve so much more than just a clap
But a long overdue pay rise
So when we're finally over all of this crap
Our whole way of living needs revised.

I hope that everyone keeps well
And we all get through this awful time
I look forward to the ringing of bells
Thinking of loved ones lost as they chime.

Davy Craig.

24/7.

Her indoors is him indoors
The tick-tock clock
They both pace the floorboards
At this new found shock
This new plague infiltrates our lands
No family gatherings, pubs or bands
Time goes by like a growing beard
As TV News feeds more plague fear
Please heed the warnings – don't ignore
Don't venture from your own front door
The N.H.S. our saviour true
For him, for her, for all, for you
Shoulders high, stands on two feet
You'll find it down…
On 'Caring Street'.

Derek B. Steel

Ague.

The fear, the fever, gripping mankind
hive minds in enlightened times
spools back as one hunkers down,
one dips into ancient wisdom for comfort
the warmth of the incunabulum
centuries-old sagacity intoned, scribed later
on palm leaves in abandoned languages
deciphered by percipient sages, a legacy
handed down by generations imbibed,
absorbed into the DNA, a rare manuscript,
an album of belonging.
Fleeting memories
cadences, rising like a lotus from a muddy
waters of a stagnant pond, revived, unwithered
old herbal remedies, that gives succour
written in the eighth hymn of the Atharvaveda

"Healing herbs …
powerful, giving life to men.
The conquering strength, the power and might, which ye,
victorious plants possess,
Therewith deliver this man here from this consumption"

Wishing the infectious virus away with Medieval
remedies, waiting for an effective vaccine.

*Note: Atharvaveda: The fourth text in the Vedas (1000-
1200 BC)*

Leela Soma.

Time

A wound, deep, scarred
not mended, fever, aches,
blurry eyed, my mind spools
sepia images, a laceration of pain
social distanced from my love
a longing to hug and kiss
her soft lips, cuddle her.

A silence, glancing at her photo
through the glass, yearning.
Solitude, would I die alone?
open to the purple skies as
bright stars twinkle mocking my hurt.

The ancient dust covers me
in a serape of memories
of our life together, halcyon days
sunshine, love, teen- glow
of childhood love and passion
under the magical moon
and time waits like sand.

Leela Soma.

Morning.

The cereal bowl, the cat stretching,
tall daffodils sway outside
purple, white and yellow crocuses
silver, gold and amethysts gems
of nature, spring has sprung.
The cherry blossoms heavy on the
tree, as the virus spreads, the world
is upside down, news pinging the
horror- another thousand dead-
lonely, wanting a human touch,
a voice to soothe, music as balm
my wild words inked on white as
unchanged world spins on its axis,
summer is yet to come.

Leela Soma.

Me Against The World.

I hail from the East like Wiseman
Vastly pandemic like bad news
Causing distress to land and seamen
Who've gathered on me to share views
It's me against the world

Yes I'm Covid
Dressed in 19 clear and strong symptoms
I'm so vivid
Irrationally destructive like bombastic atoms
It's me against the world

Religiously, I'm defined as tribulation
Or maybe the wrath of God
Luring Popes to burning incense as eradication
Hoping that "I", away they can goad
It's me against the world

I'm the new and old subject in education
Now that i had all institutions locked down
So students would read on their future's eradication
As I put all of their dreams down
It's me against the world

Scientists gathered around from every city
Trying to define a tackle on me
But I've injected the economy with paucity

Now short are the resources and now the real scientist is me
It's me against the world

Yes I'm Covid
Devourer of the future
Devouring the weak like a vulture
I'm waiting for a war
That's why I'm dressed in my 19 symptoms couture

Jay Sonnets.

Without My Furbabies.

Without my Furbabies and daughter I'd be in the canal by now their holding my depression at bay a bit, I will forever cherish the word freedom. ❤

Cat Corbally.

Reply To Ruby.

Everyone needs someone, even loners if they care to admit it.
Never easy. Windows can be cleaned, just carefully reach
out. House can be cleaned. One room per day. Can you drive?
Are you mobile? Walk, cycle. Get exercise. Take this
opportunity to notice the little things. Earth's psyche is under
scrutiny and we're the psychologists & therapists. I'm in a
reflective mood. No bad thing. In same furrow as others.
Beautifully cold.

Meek.

The Shelves Wiped Clean.

Pasta
Toilet Rolls
What the Fuck!
People get a grip
For the vulnerable
Lonely
Be kind
Where is our community spirit?
We are all in this together
The world's gone mad!
I'm just trying to do my job!
What with all the panic buying
We are all afraid, upset, freaking out.

Written by **Carol Allan**
19/03/2030

A Little Prick.

And now we can't go abroad.
And we can't just stay here
While the fresh food runs out
And we cower in fear

We watch resources run out
As our bridges are burned.
Rent our infrastructure out
Tell me what have we learned?

These people haven't a clue
These people haven't a soul
And they won't know what to do
When they relinquish control

The ones who set this shit up
Have already lost their nerve
And when the foolish wise up
They'll get just what they deserve

They gave us our right to choose
We chose to give up our rights
And then they neutered the news
And muzzled its bite

The rampant greed on display
With every nose in the trough
And if we do as they say
We'll be completely cut off

Put to the sword by our inbred overlords
Finally getting their own way
Now we're all ill they're going for overkill
But some of them are going to pay.

Jim MacKellar.

A Private Message From Davy Shared.

No problem, Meek. We're coping fine, at the minute. Think I had it in February, couldn't breathe, with a temperature etc and had to go hospital. OK now, but just hoping that's it over, as I don't want my son to get it, as he has an extremely rare breathing condition. Can't worry about it, just being vigilant. Good luck with everything!

Davy Craig.

Scared.

YOU WERE RIGHT TO TELL ME THERE WERE NO
MONSTERS IN MY CLOSET MOMMY
NOTHING HIDING UNDER MY BED
THE BOGEYMAN WON'T HURT ME MOMMY
BECAUSE WHAT WILL HURT ME KILLED HIM DEAD!

Tyhe Paul Egar.

It's Just Over There.

From a distance you would think it makes no sound at all
But how wrong you would be.
It moans and howls, screams and wails, cries and cracks!
You would think it alive, from a distance.

From a distance you would think it beautiful, it was once
All blue and green it was.
Oceans of freedom and starlight wonder and dreams!
You would think it wonderful, from a distance.

From a distance you would think it vast, but not at all
Its tiny ideas blinked out many years ago.
Gone by like the giants who once stretched across its sky
It was a world, from a distance.

Of what do I speak?
It's just over there...

Tyhe Paul Egar.

Good Luck.

As a conclusion I can say that people forget about their prime instinct - fight for your existing in the Universe! They eat too much, drink, smoke, do not fast, reduced physical activities. As a result Nature challenges them from time to time. The strongest will survive! The weakest would die. Live it or hate it it's the rules of existence; we should be in tune with the Universe!

Maliny van der Mysteries.

How Predicable Was Ernest!

"When spring came, even the false spring, there were no problems except where to be happiest. The only thing that could spoil a day was people and if you could keep from making engagements, each day had no limits. People were always the limiters of happiness except for the very few that were as good as spring itself."

E Hemingway

Ernest Miller Hemingway (July 21, 1899 – July 2, 1961) was an American journalist, novelist, short-story writer, and sportsman. Notable awards: Pulitzer Prize for Fiction (1953); ... Born: July 21, 1899; Oak Park, Illinois, U.S
Died: July 2, 1961 (aged 61); Ketchum, Idaho, U.S
Ernest Hemingway bibliography · Iceberg theory · Ernest Hemingway House

Submitted by **Maliny van der Mysteries.**

2020 Ant Army.

69

I just crushed twenty ants,
Crawling along the floor.
They were heading up the stairs,
All clambering for the door.

Roll upon roll,
Their selfish greed,
Finding what was never there before.

Alex Hughes
FRI 19:25

It's A Tough Old Choir.

It's a tough old choir,
strings, are peddling along,
Drums and percussion too, the choir master can't keep up,
what is a man to do?

It's just a shame the choir has gone,
And seems to leave us all alone.

Alex Hughes
March 2020

Michelle's Collage.

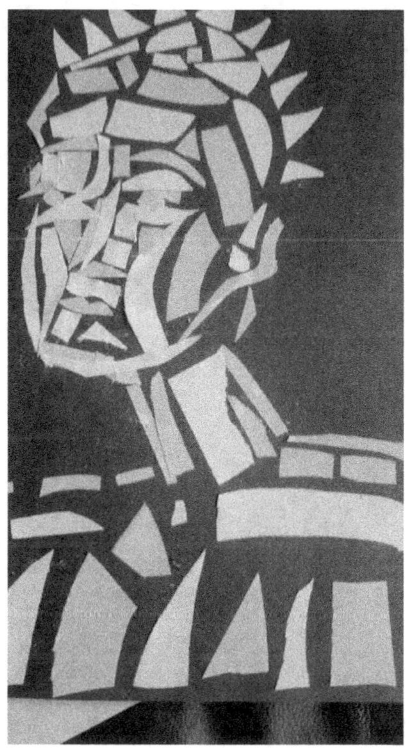

Michelle Carr.

Reply From Tyhe Paul Egar.

That's fantastic! Thank you too, I'm more than happy to be involved in something like this. If I can help at all please reach out

Tyhe Paul Egar.

Reply To Tyhe Paul Egar.

*It's just bringing us (fleetingly) closer together. Those of us
who make it through will soon forget and resume our old
ways.*

Meek

Quarantine Overtime.

"My minds doing overtime in quarantine since losing a neighbour recently. Also the people in my shops obey the 6 ft. mask floor ruling at shop entrance and checkout but not always in the aisle ."

Over-played songs
over-vacuumed carpets
over-cleaned cupboards
I'll need to replenish
my stock
off I'll trot
to those well
needed shops.

Shop floors are all masked
with six feet away tape
stick to the rules
they must be obeyed
you may now take your
trolley it's been
treated with
disinfectant spray
I have my own
hand sanitiser
anyways just in case

oh there's something
I think I might need
those tangerines
without any seeds
is that man coming
my way oh no
I can't breathe
Just in case he
Coughs or Sneezes
I don't want to
catch Covid
phew that was close
please stay out my way

Oh look in this section
I could by some
more books to read
when I don't want to cook
I could really lose myself
in a good story
an empty shelf here
an empty shelf there
no toilet rolls no bread
no baked beans or milk
where goes the meaning
to the word share ?

Here is this section
has something I
need rice pudding
some chocolate cake
now I don't need to bake
one tin of custard and
a block of cheese
and some trifles please.

At the checkout
It's masked just
the same
as at the door
when I came in
I'll wait in the
Masking tape line
good it's six feet apart
then I'll have my time
to unload and pay

Please make pay with
your bank card
sorry we don't mean
to be harsh
as we don't want
your dirty old cash

please do call again
and have a nice day
as in good health
we will bid you will stay.

Katrina McKeown.

A Story In 3 Photographs.

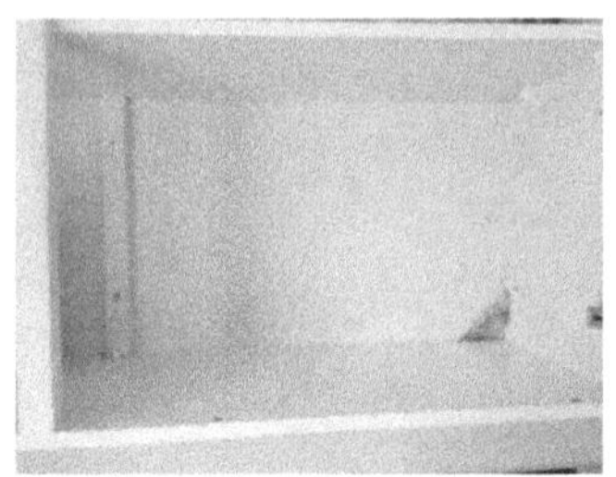

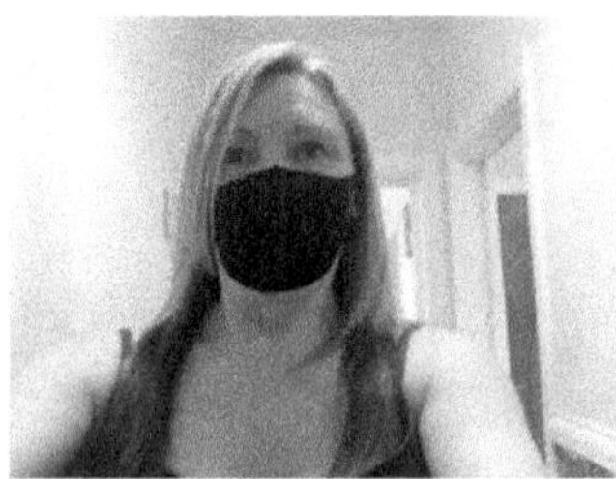

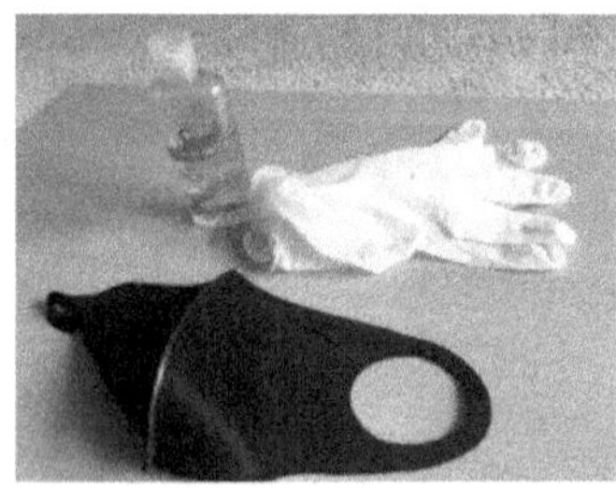

Katrina McKeown.

Erik's Perils.

When Corona Is Over, Let's All Be:-
Gentler/Kinder/Politer/Savvier/Smarter/Friendlier
Richer in our personal wisdom
Healthier in political discourse
Better in ourselves, more grounded in what matters
More connected to loved ones and to all strangers
Aware of frailties, shortcomings amid life's dangers.

by **Erik Zoha.**

Sue's Eulogy.

You are one of the coolest and interesting people I've met in a long time. (Apart from David) when you sent me the message above I thought I couldn't contribute. But my life hasn't been a quiet one so I'm certainly going to write a short piece. Even last night I'd to go to a neighbour and drop something off. I'd to wear a bloody mask and when I left and jumped over the wall, I miss judged it and skint my knees 🦵🦵

Sue Cooper.

Paul Gallagher's An Honest Account.

An honest account of thoughts, guess we've all got our own, trying to make sense of it all, the crime against the wild and beautiful, where boxes are put for us to be picked out pruned back and planted in order selected for the tidy garden the spirit less lays beneath the shady tree to grow to be cut back to grow to be cut back to be cut back to be cut back!!! 😎

Paul Gallagher.

A Bit Of Haiku.

Corona virus
Holding the world to ransom
At least it's not war??

Corona virus
The world's coming together
At least there is peace

Corona virus
When this crisis is over
I hope the peace lasts.

Ali Paterson Archer.

Corona Exhortations.

(BJ points to corona growth
trajectory on his chart):
'Flatten that sombrero!
Crack on!
Knuckle down!
Pull together!
Blitz spirit!
WASH HANDS!
Bag it, bin it -
That way we'll win it!
STAY HOME -
(Or more will die)!
Send corona packing!'

Erik Zoha.

Corona Influencers.

We've got the Green Goddess,
And Joe Wicks doing physical jerks;
Myleene helping music notation,
Vorders aiding maths computation;
LFC's Ox/Perrie, competing physical jerks,
Plus NHS staff to stop virus getting worse.

Erik Zoha.

Elvis Came To Me In A Dream.

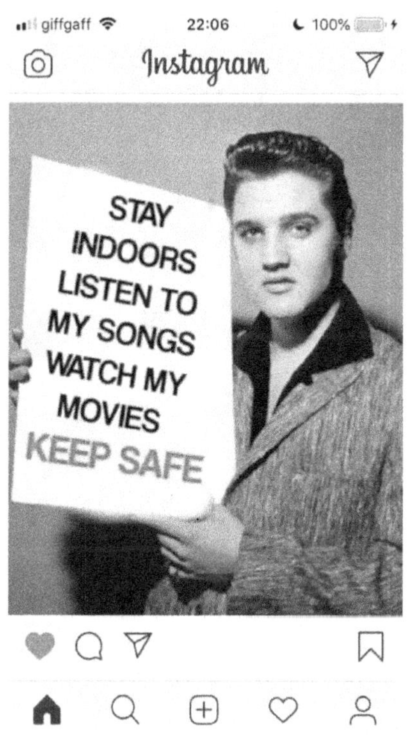

Katrina McKeown.

Falling Through Space.

Falling through space
Not sure you can trace
Where my footprint was before

Gave it my best
Passed the test
Doesn't matter any more

What I saw and thought
Can never be bought
Remember that

Lorna Kerr.

A Virus At The Door.

Knocking at our door - a virus,
Let the world admire us.
Fought a six-year battle and won,
Peace was not valued by everyone,
Tears fell into the river of despair -
Too many loved ones no longer there.
Mother cried, son went off to war,
Children waived goodbye from the door.
Who would return, who would fall?
The left-behind waited, backs to the wall.
Machine guns, bombs, rockets, direct hits,
Shrapnel, explosions, fires, blitz,
Came through a crisis worse than this,
Lived through years of peace and bliss,
Came an enemy to confine us -
Strength of character to define us.
Tough and resolute we must stay,
Victory coming soon on a bright day.
Knocking on our door - a virus,
Let the world admire us.

Rosetta Muscatt.

*Poem by Rosetta Muscatt. Age 89. Lives in Bushey. Grew up
in Notting Hill area. Worked as a secretary and a full-time
Mum. Was happily married for more than 50 years.*

Thoughts From A Surreal World.

Hello walls
Hello windows
Hello fridge
Hello cooker
How are you all today?
No different to yesterday I guess.

Remember that saying if walls could talk?
If only they could at this time.
I have a zillion things to do
I could do them today or maybe tomorrow or even next
week.

Worrying about friends with anxiety
Questioning my own sanity
Is this real or just a bad movie?
Numbers on a screen are not real people until someone you
know is snatched away.
My Christmas card list this year could be even shorter
Maybe I won't be here to send any
Keeping positive is so hard, but I must try
All I seem to be saying is BE SAFE
I hope as many of us as possible can be.
Must go and check how the kettle and toaster are doing.
BE SAFE.

Amanda Austin.

A Thought During Lockdown.

I was brought up as a Catholic, during the 70s and religion
was a big thing in my family, community and schools, but
various things made me sceptical, from around the age of ten
and I stopped believing in god, or any higher being after
seeing the Pope. That's another story, but something else has
lead me to further confirm this:

If god created everything, then he/she/they'd surely be able
to see into the future and know everything that's going to
happen, especially with what's going on in the world, now.
OK with that?
OK

Therefore, I've been thinking a lot, recently and have come
to the conclusion that the design he/she/they've made of a
certain part of the male anatomy, has not been made to
purpose:

The Willy.

He/she/they must have known that men would eventually
not just pee in the open, on a tree, or in a field, or even out of
windows onto unsuspecting passers-by, but, in the last couple
of hundred years, into a urinal, or toilet. God should,
therefore, have borne this in mind when designing the Willy,
or, at the very least, watched future episodes of The Great

Pottery Throw Down, to get tips from the design of teapot spouts, when designing the male member.

Due to this lack of foresight by the Supreme Being, men have to try and pee into a bowl, without splashing, when he/she/they could have changed the speed of flow for one. The major problem, though, is that even when being extra careful, the final drips come down the end, like pouring from a badly designed cup, not a fit for purpose spout and leave unnoticed drips on the floor, which need to be wiped and cleaned up, either by the vigilant urinator, or, in most cases, by the next person to come to use the loo, more often than not an angry wife, thereby causing more arguments and bad feeling.

I rest my case!

Davy Craig.
March 2020

Under The Darkened Sky.

From under the darkened sky, in the heart of the storm applause erupts for the heroes of yesterday, today and tomorrow.

Cheers for the heroes whose hands hold our lives, the people who take us through the dark and bring us back to the light.

Under the darkened sky. We see the end of a long trek. A journey the world united in. A journey with many stories, many tears.

All the lives clap in unison for the heroes who help us feel better, who help us through the storm and allow us to live our lives.

Under the darkened sky we win.

Ross Wilcock 2020

Bubble.

as I sit in my house
our own little bubble
I watch the kids
noticing it's Lily
who causes the most trouble

I think of the world
as it is right now...
going outside?
I don't know how

as each day goes by
we're driven a little more crazy
some may look at us
and think ha how lazy

but we do lots of stuff
arts and crafts with lots of huffs
reading and writing
Lilly keeps biting
Tyler's a maths fanatic
"what's 10x10"
of course one hundred
mummy can't keep up
how does he do it she wonders

we've had lots of deliveries
of food supplies
from amazing family
thank you guys

please everyone
keep one another safe
it won't be long
'til the world's a better place
We're all in this together
our country is one
stay home as a household
and have some fun

when this is over
Stephen and I will get wed
'til then stay home
go to bed

Kelly Greenhouse.

Isolate.

a poem a day
will take my worries away
write it all down on a piece of paper
then look back at it all them years later
laugh the fact we all became clean freaks
yet couldn't kiss each other's cheeks
you'll see how we took some time
making sure our loved ones were safe and fine
and our sadness at the many who lost the fight
because of this nasty virus that's taken flight
our life has become a bad nightmare
but we're realising just how many really care
and when we finally see the other side
we'll then realise it's just a shit rollercoaster ride
but for now run and hide before it's too late
stock up on loo roll and go isolate

Kelly Greenhouse.

Bra Masks From Debi & Carol.

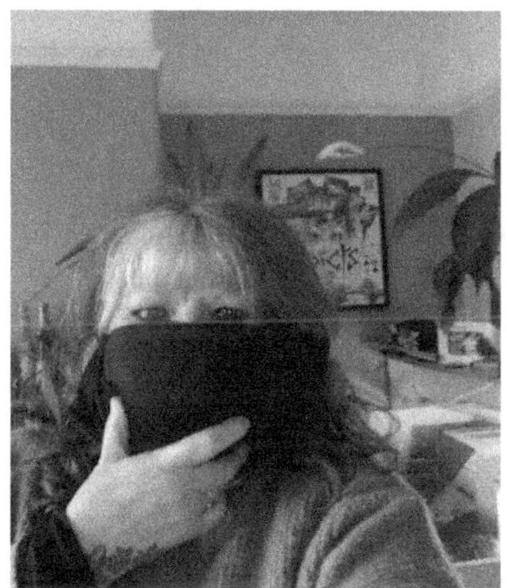

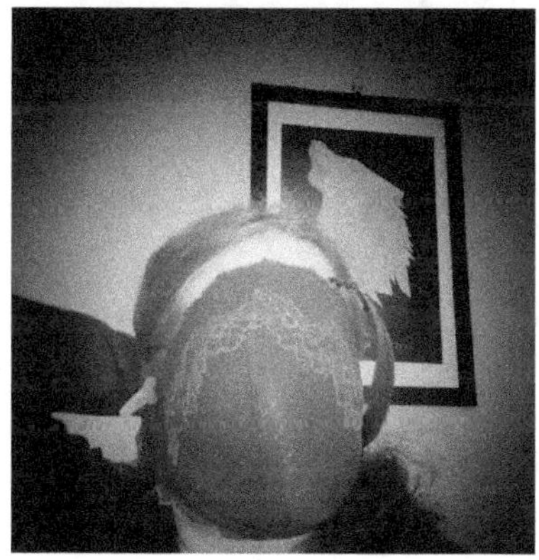

Anon.

This Time Tomorrow (Complete).

So sad to be leaving
But glad to be going home
This time tomorrow I'll be gone

Feels like it's the end
Like I'm losing my best friend
This time tomorrow you'll love someone else

So out of place
In these new surroundings
This time tomorrow you'll be more familiar

Much slower than usual
Acclimatising to this heat
This time tomorrow you'll be used to it

So take my hand
Look into my eyes
Walk a while with me
See the sunrise
See the sunrise

Surprised to see you here
Especially after yesterday
This time tomorrow I'll be missing you

Go inhale the skyline
Like a phoenix rising
This time tomorrow you'll be somewhere else

Time to scale the heights
To draw a veil across the night
This time tomorrow you'll feel different

You're making waves again
Just for the sake of it
This time tomorrow love comes home

So take my hand
Look into my eyes
Walk a while with me
See the sunrise

Take my hand

Look into my eyes

Walk a while with me

See the sunrise.

Meek

The Lull.

Suppressed anxiety building, news that awakes clarity to
confusion. The lull panic in a heartbeat. Neighbours rise to
cheer our heroes welcomed. The lull depression wages low
upsetting, survival needs becoming. The lull the calm before
the storm rising!!!!

Paul Gallagher.

Life Lesson.

Cradle to grave
In the blink of an eye,
You wail for life and then you die.

We are a mere blot on the slab,
We hurt, we heal
And pick the scab.

All about choice,
which path we take,
I hope for you
The right one make.

Alex Hughes.
1st April 2020

Risen.

Did the earth stop spinning?
Going round the bend,
Did the son not rise this morning?
When will it ever end?

Our hopes for our future,
Are all up in the air,
Or is it just reality that,
Some don't even care.

The plants they keep on growing,
Why can't we do the same,
And learn to love each other,
Alas, it's just a shame.

One day the bell will toll,
It will be the perfect day,
It will last and last forever,
We'll join and sing our all.

Alex Hughes
1st April 2020

FRUSTRATED!

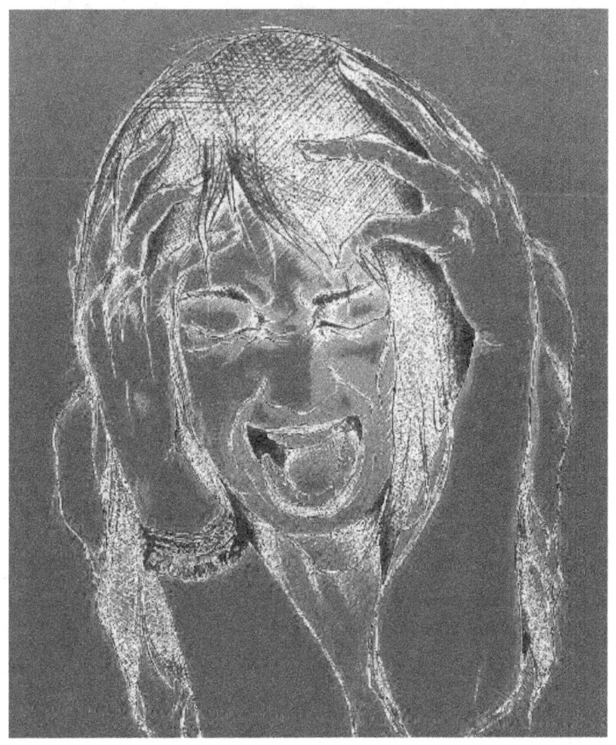

Dave Jay Coutts.

Here I Am.

Here I am sitting alone just waiting on my Friends to come!
They never do so my eyes are stuck like glue, absorbed upon
the silver screen; it seems like ages since I put the kettle on
only been two minutes now another minute's gone!!!! Just
another day, it's just another day. It's just gone nine the post
it's spot on time bet the milkman's only left a pint another
grey day there's nothing left to say, absorbed upon the silver
screen, still seems like ages from I put the kettle on only been
two minutes now another minute gone, just another day it's
just another day!!!! 😎

Paul Gallagher.

Essentials.

Yup it is, never seen nothing like this in my lifetime, I'm grounded for 3 months due to diabetes, only meant to leave the house for essential stuff or a bit walking at night ...life ain't good these days wish I could go back to the 70 and 80s...

James Molloy.

The View From A Bunker

All of us alone in our bunkers
awaiting the bombardment
Some hunker under desks
while others gaze at the sunrise
from their roofs.

John Roche.

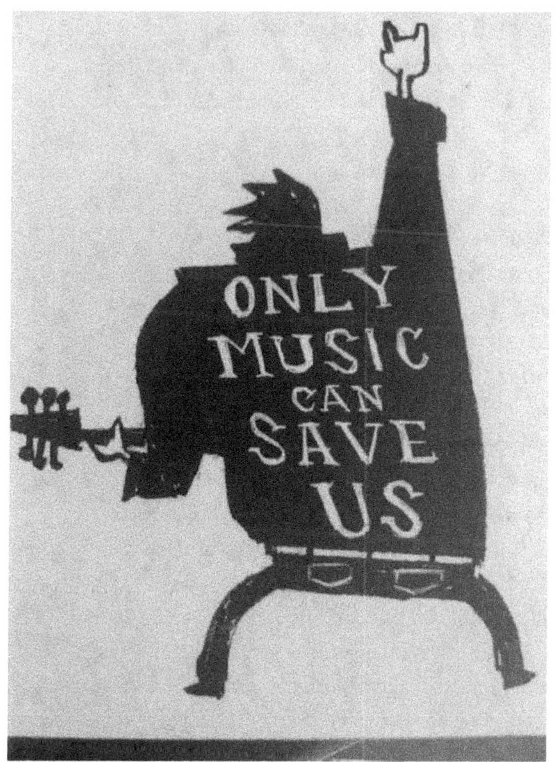

Dougie Smith.

The Corona Virus Blues.

I woke up this morning, had a tickly cough
I got a cup of coffee and I laughed it off,
Even tho I had a fever, and I felt hot and confused
I think I may have contracted
The corona virus bloody blues

I'll have to stay at home, and watch crap tv
Isolation madness that'll soon be me
I'm going crazy, and with everything to lose
I think I've definitely contracted
The corona virus bloody blues

Watching on the telly, I see there's no loo roll
We canny wipe our arses and the girls can't wipe their hole
We're going mental, and it's shortening my fuse
Because I think I've contracted the corona virus bloody blues

The wife was feeling horny; she's got a lovin heart
And then she just remembered it's two metres apart
I'm feeling cheated, and I think I'm gonna spew
I've got a feeling I've contracted the corona virus bloody
blues

This thing is getting serious, the rules we must comply
Or some of us will get a fine and some of us may die
It's getting scary, and I don't know what to do
I've definitely contracted the corona virus bloody blues

I told my wife to don, her nurses uniform
She looked at me suspiciously, coz this is not the norm
Ok baby, she winked and blew a kiss an I said
There won't be any hanky-panky
I'm sending you to Tesco for bread

I've got the coughin and the spluttering
Afraid it's make me stuttering
The two metres apart
It's breaking my heart

The stay at home and watch tv
It isn't very good for me
I'm now in the pervert club
A member of the porn hub

I'm asking myself why
It's coz I don't wanna die
Please don't let me contract
The corona virus bloody blues.

Dougie Smith.

Angels.

Hard to believe what's happening
Our worlds a different place
Everything we took for granted
Us, the human race
Now we have a challenge
Together we all stand
At war with an invisible force
In each and every land

Our ace is not a bomb now
Or a tank or plane or gun
It's angels that's our ace now
Trying to save us, every one

Never will so many, owe so much to so few
It's time we recognised them, for taking care of me and you

They don't get paid enough you know
And we know this must be changed
By politicians who are rich, and selfish and deranged

When the sun rises in the sky and this pandemic's done
NHS staff, care workers too, each and every one
You should get your medals, and a hefty bonus too
From us, your loving grateful friends
We think the world of you
If there is a god then let us pray

To the heavens up above
And thank him for his angels
Sent down to us with love.

Dougie Smith.

Sean's Post.

As I left the building both their peripheral vision saw me. Unusually today, what with the disease in full pelt, I foolishly expected some form of acknowledgement, us being of the same species, on the same side of the pavement, at the same time. However both their eyes simultaneously averted downward. She, in her tilted beret and crimson lipstick, smiled as though they were in conversation. His stride quickened as she elbowed him toward the far side of the pavement and he naturally responded, like a horse being told 'giddy up'. Their movement looked almost synchronised, choreographic, they were working together, in step, to keep themselves safe, abiding by the Government lies and completely unaware, they were already infected.

Sean Conroy.

I Remember As A Kid.

I remember as a kid, mongrel dog's roaming the streets in packs, mating season, every bitch tied to a male.
Distemper! Parvo Virus was thrown into the packs by Mother Nature, the packs became few the few became two, then the owners of one saw sense.
I don't see this no more! A lesson learnt for all,
Control what you have or pets are no more than well have nothing smile or cuddle.
Sunshine please weave, pure air hard to find yet I've breathed you in places to long to describe, my most precious time's, alone among the barley with pockets empty of silver or pound, my dog at my side with an exited eye riddled with adoration, to look to the clouds as the little burn sings and the Genny Wrenn Bob's his tail.
Sit for a while maybe shape a wry smile then throw it all into the stream, dust yourself down and head of for home 2020, there's no one around.
And yet man survived the last! X

Doug Molloy.

I wrote this wee short story just now, think it's maybe not the best story in the world but was just trying to pay a bit of a tribute to all the frontline workers that are out there doing all they can for us under extremely dangerous conditions. It's called A New Day.

A New Day.

Harry woke up, he hadn't slept too well, he had had another nightmare.

It was October 2022 and he was still adapting to the new world.
He lay and thought about the friends he had lost, and felt grateful he hadn't caught the virus.

Are you going to get up? his wife Alana shouted from downstairs, I'm away to work, Alana worked as a nurse at the local hospital and was one of the many nurses who were awarded the Victoria cross for her bravery during the pandemic, she worked 16 hour shifts for 5 months, putting herself in the front line as did her colleagues in the forth valley hospital, knowing that she could contract the deadly disease at any time.

Harry got up and went downstairs, he looked out his back window and saw another pile of chestnuts had fell from the huge tree on the other side of their fence. He loved Autumn time, it reminded him of the old days. Collecting cheggies at Bellsdyke hospital with his dad.

Half an hour later he was out on his daily walk into town, he hadn't worked since the trouble; his company had laid him off with no wages and no warning. Harry struggled with the memories he had and how he hadn't got the chance to say goodbye to his Father and his Aunt and many friends.

He was ready for his coffee this morning and jumped up the three steps of his favourite cafe, cheers, it used to be one of the Wetherspoons chain, but they went into liquidation the previous year, the whole town boycotted them, Karma, Harry had said to josh, his mate who worked in the joint.

I'll have my usual please he shouted over to Gabrielle the waitress, and a roll on square sausage please. Gabrielle was a stunner and maybe one of the reasons he used the place, he would never cheat on his wife but it didn't hurt to look.

The news was on as he waited on his coffee, the former prime minister had been sentenced to 5 years imprisonment for corruption and collusion with a Russian spy and a Chinese diplomat. Hell mend you, he muttered to himself.

The guy sitting next to him at the long breakfast bar, asked if he had a light and Harry replied that he didn't smoke. They idly chatted for a while and Harry found out the chaps name was David and he was the owner of an English engineering firm that had just been re-awarded a contract at the nearby petrochemical refinery. Harry had said he was trying to get back into work.

David was saying that this was them just getting back to begin the contract that was stopped because of the global pandemic. He had been in digs, and his family were with him when the first victims of the corona virus fell ill.

David's wee girl had been infected and almost died, if it hadn't been for one of the nurses who acted quickly and had young Dana hooked up to a respirator as soon as she was in the ward. David and his wife hadn't been allowed into the hospital and the nurse had stayed at Dana's bedside for days until she pulled through. Dana was in the next bed to an older man who was struggling; the nurse kept on crying and told Dana that the man was her father in law.

Harry stared at David as though he had seen a ghost, he brought out his mobile phone and scrolled through his photos, he showed David one of the photos and then it was David's turn to stare at Harry. "How did you get that photo?" he asked....
It was a photo of his daughter, sitting up smiling after she had pulled through

Harry replied.... my wife took it, she was the nurse that saved your daughter, and it was my Dad that passed away in the next bed.

David embraced Harry and they shook hands firmly. Would you like to come and work for me? Harry accepted and half an hour later was on his way back home thinking about his fateful morning and thinking about his beloved father who hadn't made it.

He had Alana's dinner ready for her coming in, she was exhausted but always managed a smile, the previous year all NHS staff had been awarded a 20% pay rise and the staff were happy, the world was a nicer place.

Harry nonchalantly said, "Guess who got a job today?" Alana looked at him, you?

Yes, and I got it because you are such a wonderful person. Remember Dana? The wee girl you guys saved, I met her dad David, he's given me a job as a driver, thanks to you.

She smiled, and said, no Harry, it wasn't because of me.....it was my team......and that's just what we do.

Harry smiled; He was a very lucky man.

The end.

Dougie Smith.

A Reply To My Pal, Scott Kellock.

Decades of austerity (poverty to you & I) are to blame along with consecutive governments. This, sadly, is the inevitable outcome. But rest assured, Scott, the millionaires and billionaires will still be raking it in. Decommission Trident for a start & redistribute the funds to where it is truly required. Is loss of life the cost to bring us, as a species, to our senses?

Meek
02/04/2020

Photograph I Took A Few Weeks Ago.

(Photo I took few weeks ago in the Dark Tunnel near Falkirk High Station. Zoom in. Free Mint Cracknel if you can spot Cornelius from Planet Of The Apes and Blakey from On The Buses.)

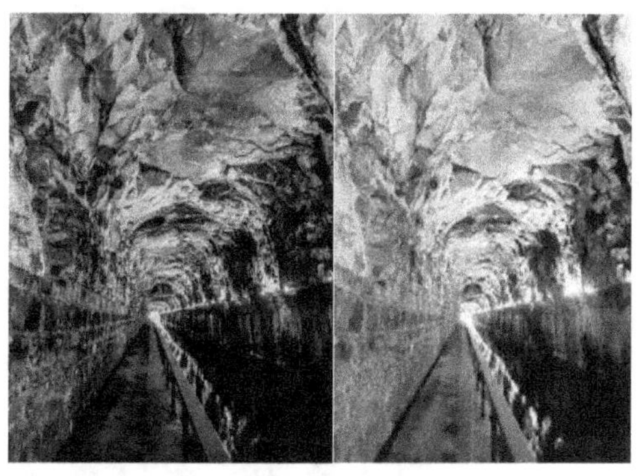

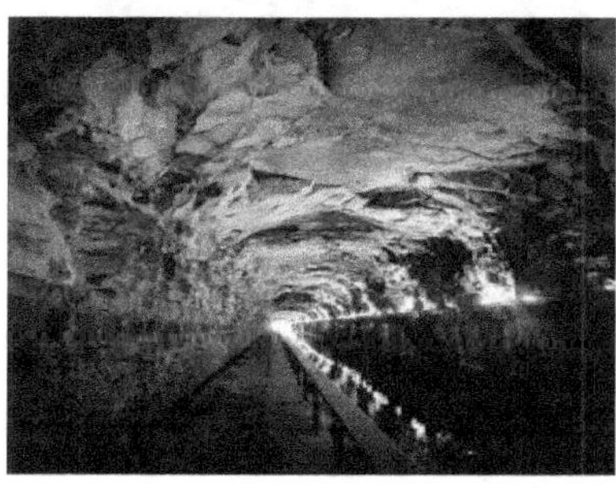

Scott Steel.

Carrying The Monkey.

The moment that I saw you,

I saw the monkey too,

You know it's always with you,

In everything you do,

Yes, I can see it smiling,

'Cause it really has a hold,

You must have it exorcised,

Well, that's what I've been told.

I wish that you could see it,

To mount a full attack,

It's already clawed in very deep,

From your shoulder to your back,

They say it is the devil's child,

They say it leads to death,

You must have it exorcised,

Or you will leave this Earth.

How long has it been with you?

When did it first appear?

Must remember time and place,

How did it get so near?

It's got a grip inside you,

It will get you in the end,

You must have it exorcised,

It's destroying you my friend.

Janette Fenton.

Touching You Touching Me.

Through the veils of sadness and the rain of tears,
Lost in this madness, frozen by the fears.
By the stream of beauty, flowing to the sea,
Near the lakes of mystery, touching you touching me.

In the arms of sorrow, again the death bell tolls,
Glance upon forever, through the window of your soul.
Dance with leaves in innocence, always to be free,
Kissing in the shadows, touching you touching me.

To drift with silent songs, a voice to melt the heart,
Bless the time together and curse the time apart.
Hand in hand to face the storm, or whatever has to be,
Hear the children's laughter, touching you touching me.

Holding on so tight, so neither of us fall.
Side by side together, when up against the wall,
We've locked our hearts forever and thrown away the key,
Love is that open hand, touching you touching me.

I face the loneliness and know you'll keep me warm,
And you'll pick up the pieces, when my heart is torn.
I give my life to you and face eternity,
Trust in love that's always, touching you touching me.

Janette Fenton.

Because Of The BEAST!

I watched the news with interest and concern,

When the Coronavirus hit Wuhan,

And the severity increased,

And more and more deceased,

Then the flights ceased,

Because of the BEAST!

Faraway people in a faraway land,

Separated by sea and sand,

And when isolation became a command,

We criticised their virus plans,

And more and more deceased,

Because of the Coronavirus BEAST!

As the death bell tolled and tolled and tolled!

I watched the naked streets,

And the laden hospitals,

And the cruel live market meats.

I watch the news with fear and dread,

As the cloud of death now chokes the earth,

And the graphs and maps increase,

To show how the spread increased,

To explain the deceased,

Because of the BEAST!

And the death bell tolls and tolls and tolls and tolls!

Janette Fenton.

Virus Sonnet 1.

I see people swarming at supermarkets
buying up everything they can carry to the car
I am aghast at their greed, at their selfishness
I see food rotting and being thrown away in weeks
I see a nurse on her way home after a double shift
clutching her last two pounds greeted by empty shelves
and I want to call them stupid, I want to rail,
I want to have them arrested and thrown into jail.

But inside me there is a screaming voice
do something, make it alright, act now
when money is the only power we have
spending it is the only thing we can do
I want to do something, I want to take back control
I want to exert my power and buy toilet roll.

Jon Bickley.

Virus Sonnet 2.

Spring is at my window and the sunshine
washes the world clean of those cloud stains
those muddy knees and boots like freshly
laundered green sheets stretched upon my bed.

The sky is watery blue, the birds watch
the dogs take their humans for a walk.
A run, a walk an escape from confines
that they still cannot get used to.

I am quarantined, Restrained by a window.
Held in a cage I stare out at the birds.
They see only the watery sky
I can hear them sing through my window
All these years we thought we owned the skies
and now I cannot leave the house for my invisible chains.

Jon Bickley.

Virus Sonnet 3.

125

Alone for a week, staring into space
I am drifting into a big nothing
a place where there is no handrail
to hoist myself up into action or attention.

Yesterday was all urgent fury, fight or flight,
and now I am in the water after
the shipwreck, a corpse bobbing on the tide
no air in my lungs, no light in my eye.

In my head I am climbing the mast
and setting sail for the promised land
my feet are floating away from my legs
waiting for something like sand
but in my heart I am beginning to see myself
as a big green fella with a trident in his hand.

Jon Bickley.

Virus Sonnet 4.

The day slips through the greasy reeds and bobs
on the lapping river, cold and silent.
Minutes seep into hours and then hours leak
into days and days go without time passing.

My boat is dissolving in the river
and before long there is now way of telling
if the boat is moving and the river is still
or the boat is becalmed on a drifting river.

Mists rise, movement ceases, silence falls,
until there is no outer world and I turn inward.
My memory offers images of torches on cave walls
potholers and divers exploring unknown worlds
but they are known in part and lovely in part
and I have all the light I need in my pen.

Jon Bickley.

Virus Sonnet 5.

The rain it rained yesterday and the rain it
rained today, the rain will rain tomorrow
ravens fly back to their high nests calling
to one another about the quiet.

The skies are clear now the people have gone.
That bedfellow that kicked all night long
has gone and now Mother Nature can share
her bed with those who want to share it with her.

Meanwhile the human flees on plague rats
gather together and reassure one
another that it will never happen
to them because they are young and special
and they grab a virus for the family
like a take away on the way home.

Jon Bickley.

Virus Sonnet 6.

I sit behind this window writing poetry
black marks appear on the page and before
you know it fourteen lines have been laid down
my little sonnet has a crown on it.

And those tall black trees at the top of the hill
stretch to scratch the clouds
like the belly of a black cat
rolling around on its back
and as the clouds glower and rage
and the rain comes down
and I catch it in my pen
and spread it on my page
and the poem takes on the personality of the clouds
and spreads all over the page
"Who said fourteen anyway
and what makes you think
you decide these things?"

My ankles swell
my waist gathers like a beach
my beard grows
til it takes over my whole face
my hair grows over my shoulders

as I settle like a house at my desk
splaying at the foundations
so I can water the garden of my poetry.

Jon Bickley.

Virus Sonnet 7.

Your long black hair was like the night sky
left upon my pillow in the morning
when you woke the two bluest stars opened
and the morning sunrise was in your smile

for the countless nights I can't remember
and the swooping love I cannot forget
swallows and martins will return one day
but they will not make their nests in my eaves

now there is such a distance between us
as if all the way to the stars themselves
and I am stranded here on the dark earth
with nothing but this desk and this pen
and this lonely night sky bereft of stars
and a sunrise grown faint in the memory.

Jon Bickley.

Virus Sonnet 8.

When you look at the stars in the night sky
you see what happened a long time ago
light takes a long time to reach my garden
it takes me longer to know what I know

If we could see our own past as clearly
not just patches of light through a shabby coat
staring at stars makes my eyes water
memories well up and swim around me

if someone asks me to describe Venus
I would point to the sky and say "Look, there"
But that would not be as she is today
it takes light so long to reach my garden
I could only say that on a good day
she outshone the moon and the milky way.

Jon Bickley.

Virus Sonnet 9.

Let there be some light said the old poet
his long beard making some kind of eclipse
and trees and birds and clouds and daffodils
the reader needs somewhere nice to stand

and there's Adam and Eve after the fall
homeless refugees and there's hunger and
poverty, betrayal and a virus
trailing after them, footprints in the sand.

"I want a poem where he loves his love,
where I can feel as if the poet is
talking to me and we like the idea
that we can see our fates in the stars
and the flights of birds, words under your breath
not exile, not pestilence, not death."

Jon Bickley.

Snowy Skies.

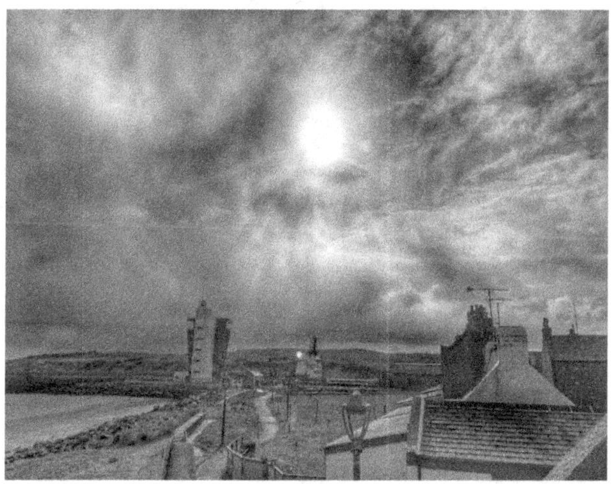

Fee Johnstone.

"The Man From Atlantis!"

"Have ye got Big Alex's number James?"
(It's Ashley in the shop)
"We've got water gushin' everywhere!"
"And we canny make it stop!"

"We've been working away at the Masons Lounge"
"And he's the man to call"
"My mate was foolin' wi' the water pipe......
And he pulled it off the wall!"

Ashley's standing at the counter
Like a begging Praying Mantis
Drippin' wet and soaked tae the skin!
Like he'd just came from Atlantis!

James is tryin' not tae laugh
(He disn'y want tae be a rotter!)
'Cos Ashley's like a drookit craw!
......Standin' in a pool ae water!!

"A' don't think Alex's the man you want
"Ye'd be better wi' his brother"
"A'l try him first James" Ashley says
"And I don't want tae tell my mother!!"

I answer my phone, and say "Hello!"
My caller`s sounding manic!
"It`s Heathers` son Ashley here!" says the voice
And he sounded in a panic!

He recites tae me his sorry tale
Of the burst pipe in the hall
How the water pressure is so great.....
It`s bouncin` off the opposing wall!!

"Don`t worry Ashley" I say with conviction
"Things will be alright!"
"It`s Alan ye need though ,a`l get ye his number!"
"He`ll soon put things right!"

Alan`s called , but alas, alack
(Ashley won`t be grinning)
`Cos Alan`s nowhere near the `Dale.......
.....He`s at his in-laws in Kilwinning!!

By now Ashley`s sloshed back up the brae
But things aren`t any better
The water`s cascading down the walls....
And he`s going to get much wetter!!

`Cos they`d found the tap to switch off the water
They gave the tap a turn
But it`s broken because it`s a hundred years old
......It`s still running like a burn!

My phone goes again , and it`s Ashley once more
"Have you got me any help?"
(The boy who pulled the pipe off the wall
Could be heading for a skelp!)

"Alan`s calling some Masons he knows"
"Richard`s trying too!"
By this time ,Ashley`d called his mum
(It was the sensible thing to do!)

The only problem being
She`d have bother drivin` oot
`Cos Heather had been in a field......
And a horse had smashed her foot!!!

"Never mind the pain yer in!"
"We`re really in a fankle!"
"There`s water, water everywhere.....!"
"And it`s well up ower ma ankle!"

Heather rushes to his aid
(Ashley`s aboot tae greet!)
A hose is soon attached to the pipe
And diverted to the street

Heather`s soon calling people she knew
A friendly plumber gent
"I`d love to help you!" The plumber said.......
.... "But alas, I`ve moved to Kent!"

The air by now, is turning blue
With no merriment or mirth
When all at once a hero arrives
......Enter, Donald Firth!

He`s the man who`s got the tools
"Right, let`s sort this pickle!"
He turns the water off out on the pavement
It soon becomes a trickle!

It was off at last, the panic over
`Ash` was soaked right through
Now of course , came the next task
There was mopping up to do!

I can only imagine (`cos I never saw it)
When the next day dawned
Instead of a brand new dental surgery.....
......It was like a boating pond!

So there`s the tale of the demolition experts
They`d certainly gave it a bash!
None more so than "The Man From Atlantis!"
Heathers` laddie `Ash`!

Big Hastie
Fae The `Dale
Dec.2008

Snapshot.

I sit here daily watching the death tolls rise
I listen to the talking heads narrating the news
They say we're in this thing together
That we must adhere to today's set of rules

I watch the images flash across the screen
I wonder if my family are aware of what's happening
We're told the same thing's going on the world over
I find it all so disheartening

I walk what were once lonely paths
I watch human beings discover their newfound joy
They're exercising, conversing and being creative
Expressing goodwill for others to enjoy

I know that some us are not going to make it
It makes me sick and it makes me sad
Our planet is beautiful yet we've taken it for granted
It's the hope of recovery that makes me feel glad

I sit here at night watching the same footage
I'm afraid that the invisible enemy may visit us
But then I'm thankful for the times we've experienced
We were born and we lived and we found love.

Meek

Memories.

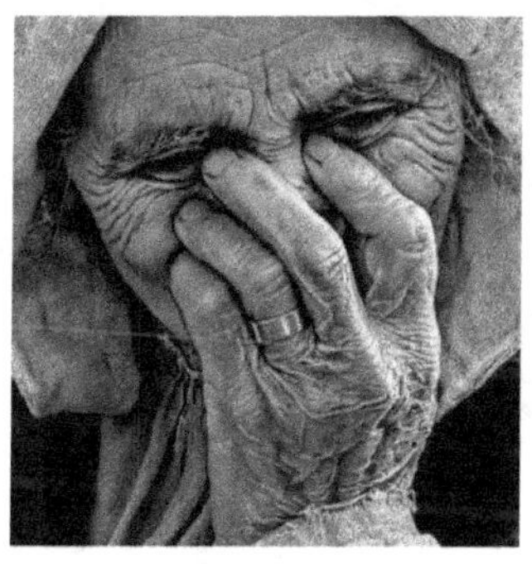

Train journeys,
The excitement,
Staying over with friends,
Sitting in a cafe watching the world go by,
Reading a book in a park on a bench,
Going to an art museum,
Any museum,
Going out for dinner,
Seeing a show at the theatre,
Oh ,how I miss a trip to the cinema!
These things will come again,
And we will make more memories.

Carol Allan 2-4-20

Some Words Might String Into Place.

I haven't written anything since the last piece I sent for Vol 13. Mind mangled manacles are strangling and distracting me from creative pursuits - but I will try and get you a piece in a day or two...if that's okay?

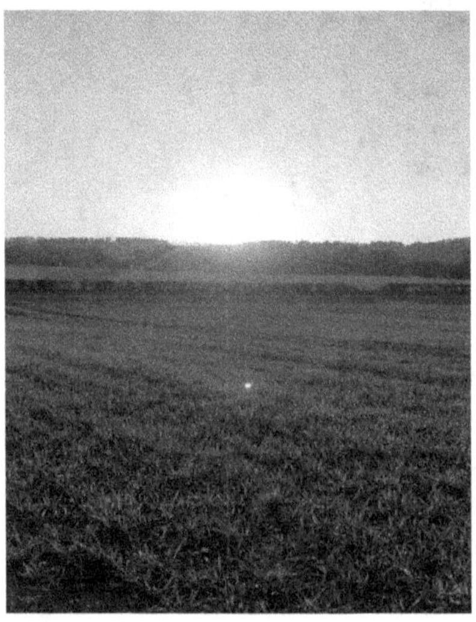

Yes, you can. I'm taking my corporeal out for a walk now, my soul is over there on the Farmer's field already... kicking stones, chatting with the hedgerows, admiring the sinking golden orb and glad to be free... So perhaps, some words might string into shape...

Niamh Mahon.

Dear Patient.

The Letter dropped ...I sanitised and opened the envelope.

Dear Patient;

Words my eyes reluctantly scan.
I make tea, sit by the window and read.
Words of caution... a list of Hearts, those born a little different
who struggled to live.
There I am...I'm on the list.
My Alien Heart that needs a machine to keep the beat while
it slowly fails
Mo the Cyborg.

Later a text.
A little hope
Lungs worse than most
But better than some
I celebrate with a stroll in the sun.

And now the call
It's Dr D ...normally annoyingly sure of herself.
But these ain't normal times.
She tries to be reassuring...telling me my follow up tests won't
happen now...
Hoping she's ending on a high she
delivers a good result from CT scan..(yay)

Then 'The Conversation'
She wants to know contents of the heart letter...she listens.
I hear pity and sadness as she gropes around for hopeful words while trying to be honest...
I feel for her...
I let her off the hook... after all it's my hook.
I dump any deference I ever had for her position...
 I say 'It's Ok Darlin... I know the score... even the smartest Cat has only nine lives ..'

This all happened yesterday. The Covid letters have been interesting to say the least. Never really thought of myself as vulnerable for all I've been a 'lifer' with heart and lungs.

"Covid letters" sounds like a spy novel 😀😀

Mo Scott.

Boathouse And Two Chairs.

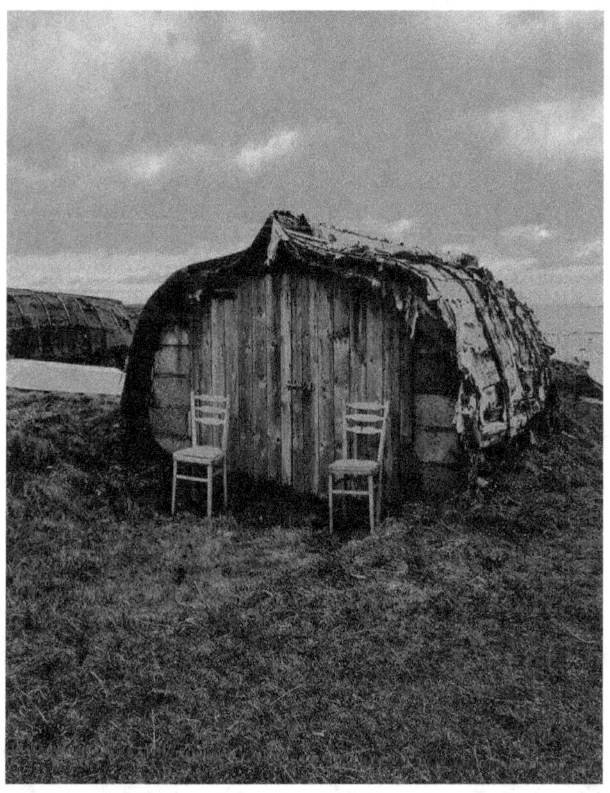

John Innes.

143

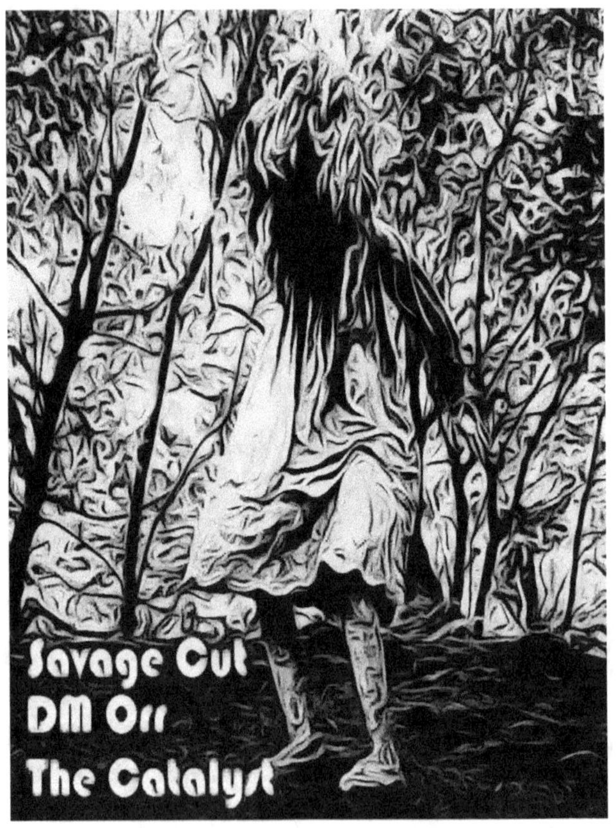

John Innes.

Applause.

How they clapped
The noise echoed through the empty streets
Emotions running high
A country comes together
For no one wants to die
Our heroes in the NHS,
And people in the shops
And lorry drivers and couriers
Out doing all their drops
A whole world now relies on you
Questions later we will ask
Right now just know we need and love you
For doing this grave task
Life for you will never be the same we hope you know
You'll always be our heroes
Everywhere you go.

Dougie Smith.

Meek's Facebook Post Regarding NHS Applause.

Pt I

I'm afraid applause won't keep our key workers alive or better equipped. They are doing a fantastic job but they always have.

Pt II

This post wasn't intended as negative. At my front door last night I experienced a sense of, dare I say, solidarity? From my neighbours and what I saw on tv screen. But I also got an overwhelming sense of futility. Is that what we, the human race, are reduced to - applauding in the face of a pandemic? Paradoxically torn and too weak to kick back against the pricks. NHS & key workers have always done fantastic jobs.

Meek.

Scott McKinlay's Post Regarding NHS Applause.

It makes me a little uncomfortable being told what to do and when! Might feel better if we all held up a sign saying "pay nurses a decent wage", but we're a nation of sheep, and we'll all go back to complying once things go back to "normal"! Teachers, the police and NHS staff don't need applause; they need to be supported by government, and paid a decent wage! Remember it's not so long ago when these same Tories, who are now telling us to applaud, are the same Tories who voted against giving, and cheered about not giving nurses a wage rise!

Scott McKinlay.

James Barney Ward's Response To NHS Applause.

I don't like being told to do what and when, but it happens at work all the time, I don't like to be called "sheepish", we all know the script what the frickin tory policies are, if I can show a little bit of appreciation to our NHS and front line workers during this panfuckindemic, then I am gonna do it from my doorstep, same as everyone else should...

James Barney Ward.

Jimmy Kellock's Facebook Reply.

You won't see me clapping m8. It's a futile gesture. Remember though these same clappers are watching to see who doesn't clap and will be making assumptions about people who choose not to. It's human nature to decry those who don't follow the norm, but if it makes folk feel better then by all means do it.

Jimmy Kellock.

The Only Place I Knew Nobody Would Be.

sick of the news making me sick
tired of the rising death count
and exhausted of people,
I went to the only place
I knew nobody would be—
no news, no chaos,
no coughing, no panic,
no food shortages,
no complaints of no toilet paper,
no empty shelves,
no sideways glances,
no people, no paranoia,
no death—
and I sat there listening
to the sound of the world slowing down.
and I watched the wind take turns
dancing with grass blades and sparrows.
and I stared at the wild pale blue sky
empty of airplanes and empty of clouds.
and the air felt clean and good.
and my mind was focused and clear.
and the gravestones
all around me
whispered: "home."

Tohm Bakelas.

Jackie Reilly's Words.

As most of you have says the NHS have always done a great job & will continue to do so after all this is done & dusted. My sister was driving through Maesteg last night at 8 o'clock on her way home from work at the Princess of Wales Hospital she was in tears at the amount of people who were out at their doors clapping it really gave her a sense of solidarity knowing that unlike this Tory government people do give a fuck. She will keep on working & trying to help patients with the virus with no PPE equipment, terrified that she catches it & takes it back to her family & knowing full well that after it's over the Tories will keep privately selling & underfunding the NHS, so for her & my own daughter (a mental health nurse) I will go out & clap, but only because I want to.

Jackie Reilly.

Next.

And the next one please. What's he done?

Missed the Thursday night national clapping for the NHS m'lud.

Any previous?

Yes m'lud. His neighbour has signed a statement confirming that he missed it the previous week too.

Was he warned?

He was issued with a letter.

Have you anything to say in your defence?

I was advised to self-isolate as I was showing signs of the virus sir.

Do you have any evidence to support this? A letter from your GP for instance?

I was told to self-isolate over the phone.

Hmmmm. A likely story. Six months picking fruit to help the nation. NEXT.

Alex Main.

Sweet Street Chalk Messages.

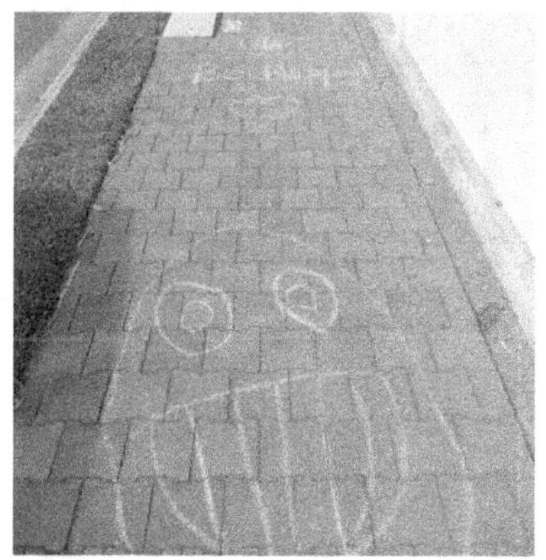

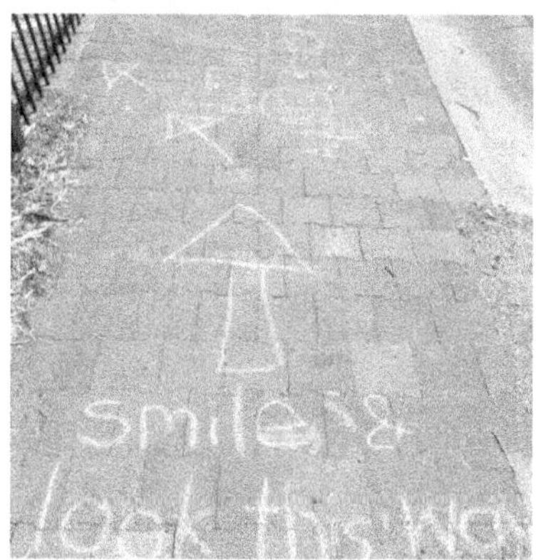

Mr Hemp.

153

Life As It Was Sketched.

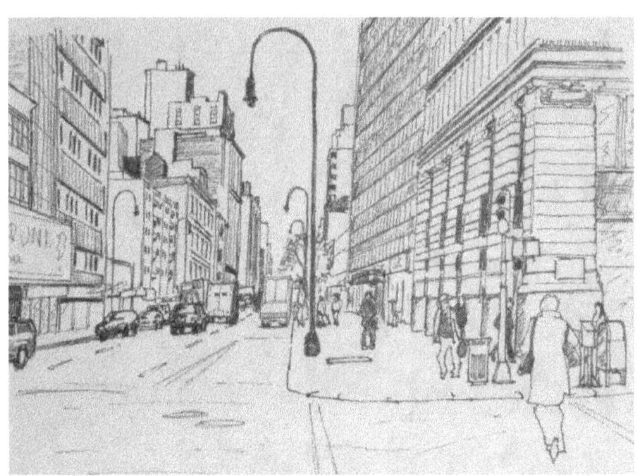

Stephen Scott.

Janet Crawford Replies.

As an ex nurse of nearly 30 years' service, I agree we have never been as valued politically as we are by the public. But, I can assure you this simple act of connection is being noticed and will be appreciated by the staff involved. I worked through Dunblane and I know I appreciated the thoughts and prayers expressed at that time, and through H1N1, I know I did and they do see and appreciate such support as health care professionals. . My lad working every hour in Tesco and trying to keep on top of Uni work virtually, my other son starting a temporary role there too. I've personally chapped the window, waved and shouted thanks to my bin men and thanked my postie. What the clapping does is show an outreach of gratitude and support, to all who are supporting us through this. What the ballot box will hopefully show in future is that we have long memories and that change is required whichever party is in power. Also, I dare BJ to sign agreements selling off our NHS. It would hopefully spell the death knell for his vicious, self -supporting brand of politics. Rant over! I apologise.

Janet Crawford.

Andy Gee Enters The Fray.

It becomes a fascinating thing watching the various ways the world is dealing with all this - the Government, having spent an entire election decrying the spending plans of the opposition, now think nothing of spending the eye-watering amounts and times it by 100 while taking the credit, and meanwhile also conveniently forgetting that if they hadn't spent the last 10 years depriving the NHS of funds and staff, that we wouldn't be in this NHS mess in the first place. That they are so woefully unprepared to protect said NHS, is a cause of major concern for everyone, but right now we have a bigger- or rather, smaller - thing to worry about, even though the average person will have one hell of a price to pay if and when we come out of this, financially, of course. But this is a matter of life and death and we do rely on the NHS and we do want them to win the war - even the people who ran them down in the first place - funny old world. Speaking of world, there are more different "cures" to all this than you can poke a pig with - in one country, you can't go out unless you phone a number to get permission while in a rather substantially larger country, travel, including flying, is still taking potential virus-carriers and catchers from one place to the next as though nothing was happening. So, bear that in mind next time you think our lockdown is a curse - it could be worse - but then again, it just might......meanwhile, on a personal basis, I miss broadcasting my weekly radio show to one man and his dog - I feel so sorry for that dog - but it's a small price to pay compared to health - this staying alive bit, is highly underrated..........

Andy Gee.

Was Not Me.

That really was not me,
What everyone could see.

That's hacked into my brain,
And make me go insane.

Perhaps it be a while,
Really do make me Rile.

Calm, slow and rest we be,
Patience it is the key.

Alex Hughes
5th March 2020

Wee Face.

I saw him peeking over the fence,
In a corner,
In the shadows
Some time hence.

It's in a breeze,
On a canoe,
Or maybe in 'awright' from a 'coo'.

Its puffed up chest,
Pointed beak,
Stick like feet
Just a tweak.

Its sun warm chest
Upon its breast,
Points us to whom,
Is in the room.

Alex Hughes.

"Suzie Q"

Raised in Brockton, Massachusetts
His parents both Italian born
Five siblings all at Brockton High
He left Tenth Grade forlorn

Ditch digger, Coalman, Shoemaker ensued
Until his draft in 43
He sailed the channel every week
From Wales to Normandy

At 5 Feet 10 and 13 stone
The world was about to see
A household name and legend
His name will never escape me

His B-52 His "SUZIE Q", albeit later
Landed sweetly on the chin," THE MONEY"
Leaving Walcott draped across the ropes
Emulating his idol Mr Gene Tunney

His relentless attacking style and will to win
Against the biggest and all the rest
Walcott, Charles, Cockell and Moore
Every man he fought came out second best

This Brockton Bomber won every fight
Despite his weight and size

Until His Cessna flight bound for Iowa
Brought about His demise

ROCCO FRANCIS MARCHGIANO
"DAVE JAY"
 ROCKY MARCIANO

Dave Jay Coutts.

I Wanna (Snapshots)

I wanna be the first and last thing you see. I wanna apply salve and/or ointment to alleviate the hotness troubling your chocolate fandango. I wanna be the alibi devoid of compromising proof. I wanna be the tiny voice through tinny walls that echo to love making. I wanna be your pluses and I wanna be your minuses. I wanna face all of your consequences. I wanna protect you when you're at your most vulnerable. I wanna be your absolute answer. I wanna be your lockdown. I wanna be the ghost that exists alongside God. I wanna play no part in faith's fear or rules. I wanna look in your mirror in the morning. I wanna press transmission low. I wanna isolate your individual virus. I wanna borrow huge amounts of printed money. I wanna affect world standstill. I wanna claim new benefits. I wanna govern future volunteer reductions. I wanna think right now and act fast and decisively. I wanna believe in unparalleled richer countries. I wanna eradicate devastation. I wanna help current diets. I wanna supper on organic sultanas. I wanna give you apples from safe refugee camps. I wanna realise the seriousness of the situation. I wanna have food. I wanna share my sherbet fizz powder. I wanna be back in the depot. I wanna rid us all of nausea. I wanna disrupt global supply. I wanna jibe at potential damage limitation. I wanna, for definite, trade free. I wanna meet the world's needs. I wanna appeal to youth. I wanna be made an example of. I wanna rock back and forth. I wanna applaud key workers. I wanna rebalance not saying a word. I wanna challenge white collar sector. I wanna reflect upon petulant monuments. I wanna be closer than two metres apart. I wanna ask straight forward questions. I wanna ease the pressure. I wanna be with you. I wanna keep myself to myself. I wanna behave. I wanna join the dots. I wanna connect. I wanna live and breathe night and day. I wanna get critical as of yesterday. I wanna hear the nightingale sing. I wanna ventilate actual figures. I wanna serve you with popcorn without kernels. I wanna be a naked astronaut. I wanna be swimming underwater. I wanna be central to the plot. I wanna eat fire. I wanna be an age time forgot. I wanna be remembered. I wanna be all the sweeter. I wanna be the scenario. I wanna be dripping wax. I wanna a sober sot. I wanna be a faith healer. I wanna be a blood clot. I wanna chill. I wanna be faster than an endangered cheetah. I wanna see the horizon's dot. I wanna be closer than nearer. I wanna unravel knots. I wanna exercise. I wanna shop. I wanna leave home. I wanna be vast. I wanna exit easier. I wanna buy a job lot. I wanna look at you differently. I wanna be locked in a freezer. I wanna find a bargain. I wanna flout rules. I wanna remain a zealot. I wanna lose control. I wanna be a diamond geezer. I wanna disperse the minority. I wanna hug a tree. I wanna creep to a higher level. I wanna choreograph a foxtrot ballet. I wanna make decisions. I wanna stay at home. I wanna learn curves. I wanna know what happens next. I wanna be too early. I wanna pray. I wanna crack down. I wanna be tested. I wanna get my hands on medical supplies. I wanna kitten. I wanna set standards. I wanna address the nation. I wanna abolish hierarchy. I wanna dissolve channels. I wanna admit

I'm afraid. I wanna believe the players. I wanna do facetime or skype. I wanna be the one who comes back. I wanna capture the lengthening daylight. I wanna listen for a delivery. I wanna read impartial papers. I wanna be lop-sided. I wanna burn limited oxygen. I wanna learn from history. I wanna process personal protection. I wanna wear a happy mask. I wanna ditch bin liners. I wanna upgrade individualism. I wanna sit here decomposing autopsy material. I wanna clutch rosary beads. I wanna hold a blade. I wanna escalate non-essentials. I wanna confront harm's way. I wanna embrace you. I wanna minimalize unnecessary Americanisms. I wanna go further leftfield. I wanna compete against the rubbish. I wanna be heard. I wanna save lives. I wanna mention the blitz spirit. I wanna be clear. I wanna be out of the ordinary. I wanna travel. I wanna switch off repeats. I wanna watch joyous updates. I wanna bend the capacity. I wanna ban judgement. I wanna notify anti-brigades. I wanna contribute to religious unions. I wanna quote sources close to the quote. I wanna do something for the high horses. I wanna say hello. I wanna holiday. I wanna stay safe. I wanna help. I wanna heed advice. I wanna authenticate documents. I wanna be the anti-body. I wanna make sure. I wanna let go. I wanna deploy standards. I wanna be a scientist. I wanna move today onward. I wanna text you. I wanna contact virtual reality.

Meek.

What Part Of This Isn't Clear?

What part of this isn't clear?

- essential supplies
- work
- medical reasons
- exercise

I don't see "kids party in front garden" on that list.

Some people don't get it.

Neil Hodge.

Scott Steel's Poster (Filtered).

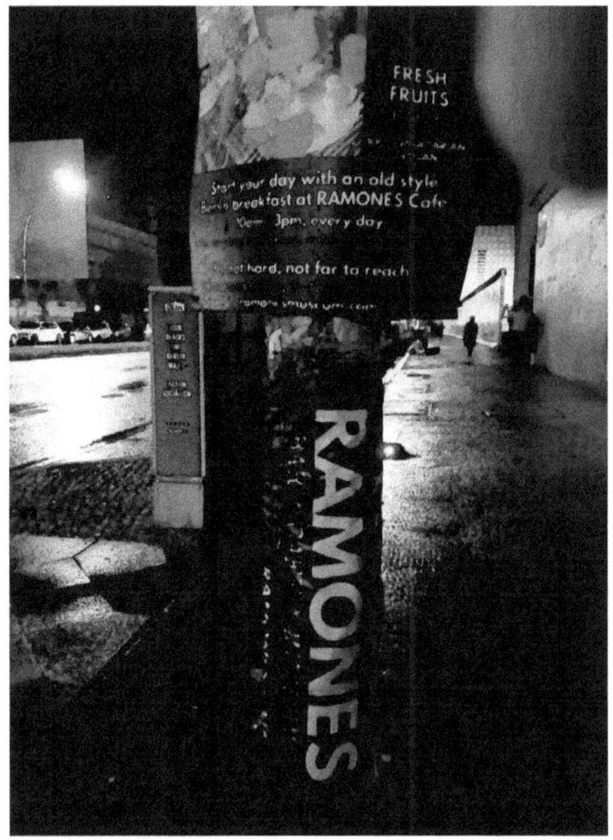

Scott Steel.

Alibi (2.22.40 Epitaph).

This Facility Is Closed read the handwritten sign, another local business run into the ground. "This was unforeseeable. This is unprecedented." Italicised for generations still to come, mentioned as an historical aside, and rammed home day after day.

We Have Ceased Trading due to the current situation. In actual fact our premises are transient. Staff furloughed. Their entitlement is less than the pittance they were paid in wages/salary. Fixtures and fittings for sale. But there's a party in full swing on the Immoral Estate.

We Are In This Together, plebs and toffs. And the ones who scoff (and cough) behind the blitz spirit pact (I mean beleaguered mentality) makeshift coffins, improvised morgues, rough and ready funeral parlours, quick and dirty services.

Amen.

Meek

AIRBORNE: The Serpent

From the Depths came the Serpent
A Silent, Sinewy embodiment of Hell
Hissing out its Venomous Lust
From Hades Deep, to ring Death's Knell!
Out Damn Creature, the Imagining's of Lucifer
A Fearful Sight, we must Repel
Kill it, Smite it, Still its Essence
Leave it Desolate, a Vengeful Shell!

Dr Ian Mowbray.

Sometimes, Neil.

Sometimes it feels like the world is falling apart around me and at other times I feel like nothing is different.

When you see upturned trolleys in Asda car park marking the correct spacing for social distancing in queues, and people shuffling between them, it reminds me of scenes from zombie apocalypse movies. Things are a bit surreal in a lot of ways. It does feel like living in several movies I've seen over the years. It's just that this one with a pretty boring script.

Thankfully, I can do my job from home with a bit of adaptation. It is keeping me so busy I probably don't have time to sit and brood on things. If I did, these words may be completely different. I'm sure my anxiety and over-thinking would kick in big time. As it stands, I'm strangely OK with the whole situation.

I'm not scared of the Virus in itself. I'm sure at some point I'll get it and just have to see how badly or otherwise it impacts me. I do fear for my folks and my in-laws though, as they are in the vulnerable category and fully self-isolating as a result. I wish everybody took the whole threat seriously though. Those who flout the guidance and think they are above it all are probably the ones who will end up passing it on to others but be Ok themselves, they think they're invincible. If only this virus could discriminate...

I'm missing live music. But that is transient, there will be rescheduled dates and new gigs to go to. My disappointment is nothing compared to the impact on others — losing loved ones, or jobs. Not being able to maintain their livelihoods, having to adapt to a whole new world. The impact on the homeless too, not just from a financial perspective with virtually no-one on the streets to stop and give them some money or some food, but from a mental health perspective. Many will be suffering anyway, but to have no-one to stop, even just for a few words must exacerbate their situation.

My biggest fear, and I try not to dwell on it too much, Steven Covey's circles of influence and concern and all that, is the impact on the world post Virus. The long-term financial impact, another Great Depression? Unemployment rising? As we come out of it, people will be encouraged to spend, spend, spend — but will we want to? Once bitten, twice shy. As I say, I'm trying not to dwell on it.

But generally, I'm in good spirits. Outside work, apart from missing live music, I'm good with this social distancing malarkey. To be honest, in a lot of ways, it is the way I would choose to live. Well, to be honest, I'd like even more of my own company, no matter how much I love my family. I like my own space. Social anxiety does have some benefits, although all this speaking to people on phones is shit. I hate speaking on the phone. I prefer written communication.

Talking of communication. The other thing that is obvious is the changing language of the country. People no longer sign off their conversations with see ya' later or cheers — stay safe is the new buzz phrase amongst other terminology.

The world has changed. Who knows what the future holds? For now though, for most, getting through until tomorrow is enough.

Neil Hodge.

My Friend.

The trip was such a sad one, there we were all set
Taking our wee collie, he's going to see the vet
We know he won't be with us when we drive back the way,
alone
And as we drive I think about the day we brought him home

This little bundle of joy, playful as a child
Whining for his mummy, and running round so wild
Wee sharp teeth and puppy breath and eyes that shone so
bright
I'm thinking how they sparkle, and how I'll miss these eyes
tonight

As he grew up and we got close, and his bark got loud and
deep
And he would aye be there for me....I'm trying not to weep
He's old now, and he's had his day, I look at him once more
My wife is holding him so tightly, I'm sure he knows the
Score

He could hardly walk, he was in pain, we have to follow
through
My wife is whispering in his ear, saying I love you
The surgery sits before us now, and Sebastian was shaking
I pick him up and in we go, my heart was surely breaking

We held him close as the task was done and his life away did
seep
He closed those gorgeous sparkling eyes and then he was
asleep
We walked away without him, we didn't say a word
The thought of life without our friend, was really just absurd

But hopefully he's somewhere nice now, running wild and
free
Over the rainbow where dogs go and happy he will be
And although I'm broken hearted, and for him it is the end
I wouldn't change things for the world; I loved him, my best
friend

Dougie Smith.

Lockdown.

Lockdown!? Lockdown! Fux Sake! Gie me a key,
So that I can escape frae ma ain companee!

Ah talked tae masel'. Ah never could hear!
Pure racket of Life drooned me oot, see, ma dear!
But noo there's nae noises from buses nor cars
Ah hear ma ain drivel - and, yayzooks, it jars!

Ah look oot ma windae for a buddy to chat
An' aw ah can see are "twa dugs" and a cat!

Tesco delivered! A man came to the door!
Posted ham throo the letterbox - nary one item more!
Then ran fur his van, like Hell was descendin' -
Not givin' a fart that he was offendin'
an auld wife in lockdown whose hair has turned yella.
"Don't like bloody Goldilocks!", I cried to yon fella.

Hairdresser's impervious. Will nut dae his duty
To transform me back tae a silver-haired beauty.
Even my dentist has closed all his doors.
My teeth are pure black - like the heads in my pores!
Nae facial fur me. Ah'm looking real ugly!
(Like the duck, not the swan) - Jings, ma jowls are juggly!

Ma TV is screamin', "Ah want an 'oor aff!"
Ah'm gulpin' the Buckfast. Ah need sumhing tae quaff!

Ma laptop's burnt oot. Pain in the Ass!
I cannae even meditate online wi' Ram Dass!

The stores are all closed. Ikea is shut!
Nae sofas tae curl oan, nor their heating to cut
ma ginormous fuel bills _ Ma Goad, aw this costs!
Ah've hud tae wear thermals tae keep oot the frosts!

However, Humanity, ah'm nae yin tae complain
Even though this infringement makes me tot'lly insane!
There are dolphins in Venice - clean air in Beijing!
Wee Greta Thunberg and her followers sing!
Such good could result, when all's done and said.
An' for me the best bit would be - not to be dead!

Sandra Alexander.

The Clocks Go Forward.

The clocks go forward,
but nothing else does
People say they have faith
in the lord up above.

I don't think there's a god.
Just nature's free will
That we sort of forgot
until it stopped us still.

We're quite alone
in our endless universe.
But staying at home,
really isn't the worst

Caring and cleaning,
learning the piano,
some like woodwork or painting
others, dreaming on the patio

It's tough in the high-rise
with too little space.
Hold close all your children
Adore their beautiful face.

It's love now that matters,
of people the most.
Please stay together,
try not to get lost.

Let go of the anger
and banish the fight
Just love your neighbour
She'll see you right.

Help the most feeble
Support the NHS
In months, maybe weeks,
we'll regain our happiness.

So, as we lose an hour,
to Spring's rain and shine
let's not lose hope, but
bless every. moment. of. time.

Michael Zur-Szpiro.

Random Thought For The Day.

Given that I, like many of us, are working from home and doing a lot of video conferencing, I am getting more and more exposed to annoying "management speak." When I did my MBA, the first course should have been "How not to talk like a twat." However, a lot of people need to go on such a course, methinks.

Current phrases that get seriously on my breasts are:

"How do you see that in your world?"

"Can you walk into that space?"

"We've done a deep dive" (I wish you would!)

And any bell end whose starts the answer to a question with "So,..."

There was an excellent comedy programme in the 1990s called "Drop the Dead Donkey", where the CEO, Gus Hedges, thought he was a management guru. His phrases were (unintentionally) funny. Such as:

"George, let's enter my workspace and create a centre of excellence."

"Can we stir-fry some concepts in the strategy wok?"

However, in the real world, we seem to have forgotten how to use language properly. It really boils my urine, and this is only the end of Week 1 of "Business as Usual via the Mac." Rant over (for now)."

Simon Rowberry.

Building Upstairs At The Anchor.

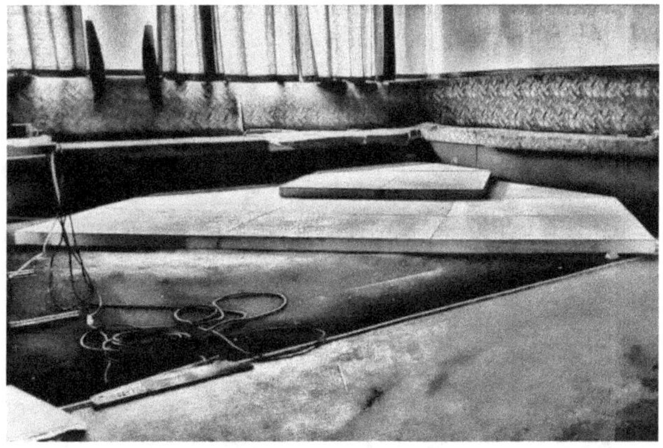

Dave Jay Coutts.

Spring Poem By Jessica Aged 7.

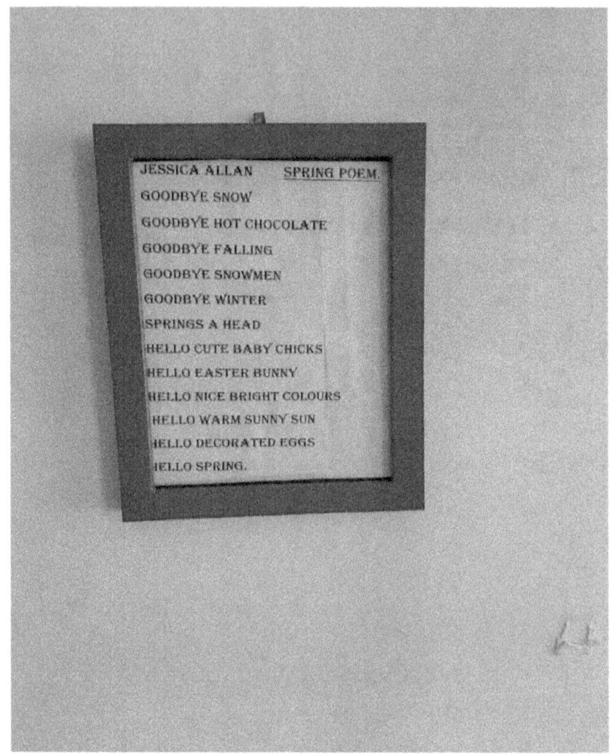

Jessica

Thanks For The Nomination, Jimbo MacKellar.

Let's do this for 75% of all suicides, that are committed by
men, too many already have been taken way too soon!
We can't keep letting this slip by us, be strong, be there for
each other and please never be afraid to speak up or try and
reach out to anyone, even myself!

John Innes.

Lynn's Post.

Didn't want to go to work today. Didn't want to go to work yesterday. Don't want to go to work tomorrow.
But I will be there till I'm no longer able and like most other folk out there who have to be there, probably well past able.
If you can stay at home and be safe, then please, do it!
Ps, I've sterilised my phone and changed my gloves. Stay home, stay safe. Xxxxxxx

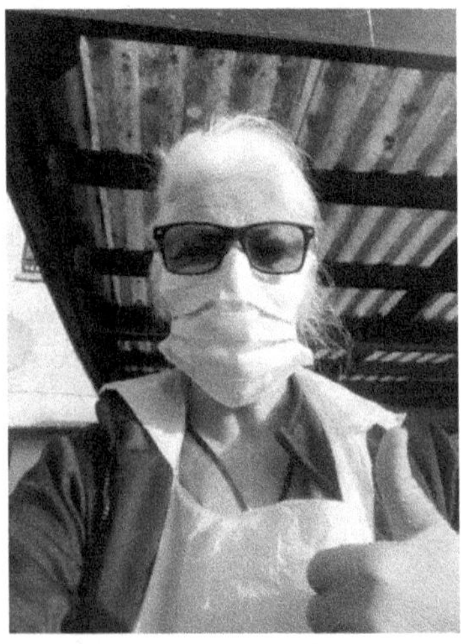

Lynn Ainslie.

It's A Family Affair.

I was born on 1 December 2019 in Wuhan, China. The exact details of my birth are unknown but my favourite version of my birth story is the one about the bat who bit a scientist at a research lab — I suppose that's the price you pay for using mammals for research.

As soon as I manifested, I knew I was destined for extraordinary things. You see, I was born into the Coronavirus family — a family infamous for reigning terror on respiratory systems.

There are more Coronavirus family members than Kardashians — that's how big our clan is. Like the Kardashians, we are a varied species, some of whom revel in the limelight more than others. Some of my more benign relatives shy away from too much controversy and are content with throwing the common cold at people. The last thing I wanted was to be common, however.

But then there's my older siblings, SARS and MERS, who aimed a little higher. Between them, they racked up around 1600 fatalities across around 28 countries. Impressive but still, they could have done better. Like that old fellow, Influenza.

I'd heard about Influenza through the virus vine — he's a notorious beast who infects thousands of people every year.

But Influenza has gotten complacent in his old age. The researchers know where they're at with him. They could probably obliterate him completely if they wanted but because he helps keep the population down, they are pretty lenient with him.

I knew if I wanted to achieve the infection levels of Old Influenza, I had to act fast; I had to find as many hosts as quickly as possible. China had been good to me and the dumplings are divine but it was time to spread my droplets and travel the world.

I relied on tourists to take me home as a souvenir for their friends and families. Never again would they complain about only getting a leaky snow globe or a spit-through T-shirt. Instead, I generously gifted them with coughs, fevers, diarrhoea and breathing problems. But my real talent lies in secreting myself inside them so they don't even know I am there. I lurk in the shadows of their lungs and watch as they unknowingly infect those around them.

I know those pesky scientists have plans to flatten my curve but there's plenty of life in me yet. I've yet to explore the coral reefs of Tonga or the white beaches of Samoa but travel restrictions are making it difficult. I need to find a way in — maybe I'll call in a favour with my old bat pals, they are such great hosts.

Perhaps I sound greedy — some have even called me a narcissist — but there's nothing wrong with being a high achiever. But you humans are making it difficult for me to attain world domination. So I beg you, humans of the world, don't burst my protective bubble just yet.

Please do not stay at home.
Please do not observe social distancing rules.
Please keep popping to the shops for a Bounty and packet of Skips.
And please stop washing your hands to the tune of Happy Frickin Birthday.
(Though if you do insist on being uncharacteristically hygienic, the chorus of I Am The One and Only will much better satisfy my ego.)

Fee Johnstone.

When.

When,
once, on the dance floor .
we elongated arms and contracted with cephalopodic joy
through the stretched beats of swung notes;

Now
here right now ,
condo-fied, recycling one's daily loops,
thicker now, precluding--like--everything that used to go on!
(out there.)
Twisting now through the company of oneself,
sometimes irksome and sedimentary,

When
once we gulped wholesale the music that resonated off our
bones
so closely we brushed the air against one another,
living as a herd, a tribe-- sentient, multi-prismed lenses.
We had drinks on tables, with maybe nachos on order

Now,
here right now,
our lone home narratives have assumed that elasticity
we once practised, uncoiling cyber limbs across the space
around us now to reach out and pluck a petal or rather the
scent of a Facebook update, oh look dear friends--rosy, rosy
hope ahead!

Our story stretches uncoiling and ceaselessly elongating,
refreshable, streaming thread-tentacles trailing downstream
from the original anchor post.
And there's a link on the home page!

Additional thoughts, accompanied by photos driven by who-
knows-what-to follow. Possibly.

Or perhaps a poem. Maybe this one:

A great exhaling contraction
tightens around our solitary bellies,
condo-fied for the duration.

Andrea Doria.

Prologue.

Goodnight,
Sister
Hopefully this isn't goodbye ......

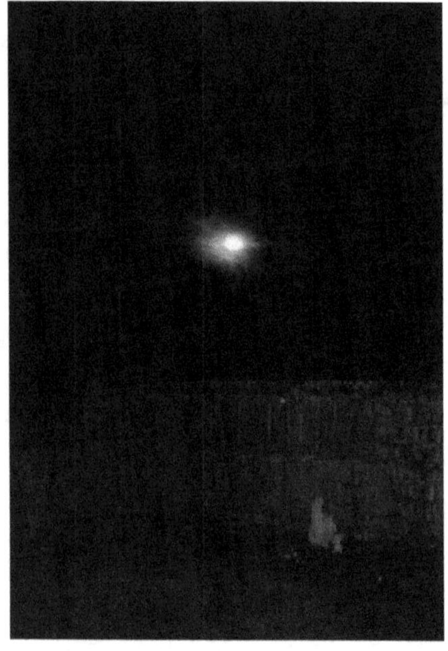

Meek.

Acknowledgements.

To everyone who contributed to this book I thank you. To the key workers during this crisis, we thank you.
Also acknowledgement to the Oxford Dictionary, Wikipedia, Google and the education system.

Meek
April
2020
x

Notes -